Chun-Su Yuan, MD, PhD
Editor

Handbook of Opioid
Bowel Syndrome

T0314399

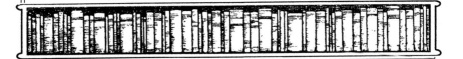

More pre-publication
REVIEWS, COMMENTARIES, EVALUATIONS . . .

"Opioids remain our most effective analgesics for many pain states, but their efficacy comes at the price of considerable acute and chronic toxicity. Much attention has been given to effects such as respiratory depression and addiction liability, which occur infrequently when the drugs are used appropriately. Much less has been written about opioid-induced bowel dysfunction (OBD) even though constipation, nausea, or ileus probably affect the majority of patients receiving moderate doses of opioids. For cancer patients and others requiring chronic high-dose opioid therapy, these effects can be enor- mously distressing and even dangerous.

This book reviews OBD from every possible angle. The chapters range from basic gastrointestinal physiology and pharmacology to clinical chapters on the pathophysiology of chronic constipation and postoperative ileus. Heavy emphasis is placed on peripheral opioid action, since much of OBD is mediated by the effects outside the central nervous system. Outstanding reviews of investigational opioid antagonists can reverse or prevent OBD while sparing central effects such as analgesia. These drugs may also block opioid actions on lymphocytes; this area is covered in a fascinating chapter on opioid-induced immunosuppression. The contributors have done a great service by bringing all of this together in one accessible volume—it will be an invaluable reference for opioid pharmacologists and clinicians who regularly prescribe opioids for pain."

Carl Rosow, MD, PhD
Professor of Anaesthesia,
Harvard Medical School;
Anesthetist, Massachusetts
General Hospital, Department
of Anesthesia and Critical Care

"Although the topic may sound narrow in scope, this book is quite broad in its appeal. The introduction sets the stage, lays out the basic physiology, and foreshadows the issues the reader will see addressed later in the book. This approach makes the book interesting for nonspecialists and researchers alike. The chapters on the basic physiology also include some practical information on opioids. The chapter on opioid-induced immunosuppression makes interesting reading and raises interesting questions regarding the other effects of opioids. The section titled 'Clinical States' is practically oriented and will be useful to anyone who takes care of patients receiving opioids or undergoing significant surgery.

Last, the book looks at two new drugs in clinical development that are both selective opioid antagonists, yet quite different. These chapters make excellent reading and provide good insight into developing new drugs. These approaches will soon offer doctors new alternatives to treating OBD in their patients."

Robert J. Israel, MD
Senior Vice President, Medical Affairs,
Progenics Pharmaceuticals, Inc.

Handbook of Opioid Bowel Syndrome

HAWORTH Therapy for the Addictive Disorders
Barry Stimmel, MD
Senior Editor

Drug Abuse and Social Policy in America: The War That Must Be Won by Barry Stimmel

Pain and Its Relief Without Addiction: Clinical Issues in the Use of Opioids and Other Analgesics by Barry Stimmel

Drugs, the Brain, and Behavior: The Pharmacology of Abuse and Dependence by John Brick and Carlton K. Erikson

The Love Drug: Marching to the Beat of Ecstasy by Richard S. Cohen

Alcoholism, Drug Addiction, and the Road to Recovery: Life on the Edge by Barry Stimmel

The Group Therapy of Substance Abuse edited by David W. Brook and Henry I. Spitz

Handbook of Opioid Bowel Syndrome edited by Chun-Su Yuan

Handbook of Opioid Bowel Syndrome

Chun-Su Yuan, MD, PhD
Editor

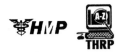

The Haworth Medical Press®
The Haworth Reference Press™
Imprints of The Haworth Press, Inc.
New York • London • Oxford

For more information on this book or to order, visit
http://www.haworthpress.com/store/product.asp?sku=5523

or call 1-800-HAWORTH (800-429-6784) in the United States and Canada
or (607) 722-5857 outside the United States and Canada

or contact orders@HaworthPress.com

Published by

The Haworth Medical Press® and The Haworth Reference Press™, imprints of The Haworth Press, Inc., 10 Alice Street, Binghamton, NY 13904-1580.

PUBLISHER'S NOTE
This book has been published solely for educational purposes and is not intended to substitute for the medical advice of a treating physician. Medicine is an ever-changing science. As new research and clinical experience broaden our knowledge, changes in treatment may be required. While many potential treatment options are made herein, some or all of the options may not be applicable to a particular individual. Therefore, the author, editor, and publisher do not accept responsibility in the event of negative consequences incurred as a result of the information presented in this book. We do not claim that this information is necessarily accurate by the rigid scientific and regulatory standards applied for medical treatment. **No warranty, expressed or implied, is furnished with respect to the material contained in this book. The reader is urged to consult with his/her personal physician with respect to the treatment of any medical condition.**

Cover design by Kerry E. Mack.

Library of Congress Cataloging-in-Publication Data

Handbook of opioid bowel syndrome / Chun-Su Yuan, editor.
    p. cm.
    Includes bibliographical references and index.
    ISBN-13: 978-0-7890-2128-1 (hc. : alk. paper)
    ISBN-10: 0-7890-2128-5 (hc. : alk. paper)
    ISBN-13: 978-0-7890-2129-8 (pbk. : alk. paper)
    ISBN-10: 0-7890-2129-3 (pbk. : alk. paper)
    1. Constipation. 2. Opioids—Side effects. I. Yuan, Chun-Su.
    [DNLM: 1. Constipation—chemically induced. 2. Constipation—drug therapy. 3. Constipation—physiopathology. 4. Analgesics, Opioid—adverse effects. 5. Intestines—drug effects. WI 409 H236-2005]
RC861.H23 2005
616.3'428—dc22

2005006939

CONTENTS

SECTION II: CLINICAL STATES

Chapter 4. The Epidemiology of Opioid Bowel Dysfunction **61**
    Ysmael Yap
    Marco Pappagallo

Chapter 5. Opioid Bowel Dysfunction in Palliative Care **69**
    Nigel P. Sykes

**Chapter 6. Opioid Bowel Dysfunction in Acute
and Chronic Nonmalignant Pain** **101**
    Keri L. Fakata
    Ashok K. Tuteja
    Arthur G. Lipman

ABOUT THE EDITOR

Chun-Su Yuan, MD, PhD, is the Cyrus Tang Professor in the Department of Anesthesia & Critical Care at the Pritzker School of Medicine, University of Chicago. Since 1994, Dr. Yuan has been conducting clinical trials evaluating the safety and efficacy of a novel peripheral opioid receptor antagonist, methylnaltrexone, for reversing opioid-induced bowel dysfunction. He has published over 150 research papers, including many articles on opioid action and antagonism of opioid side effects.

CONTRIBUTORS

Eric J. Bieber, MD, Chairman, Obstetrics and Gynecology Medical Director, Women's Service line, Senior Vice President Geisinger Health System, Danville, Pennsylvania; e-mail: <ejbieber@ geisinger.edu>.

Thomas A. Boyd, PhD, Vice President, Preclinical Development and Project Managment, Progenics Pharmaceuticals, Inc., Tarrytown, New York; e-mail: <tboyd@progenics.com>.

Cormac Fahy, MB, BCh, FFARCSI, FANZCA, Visiting Associate, Department of Anesthesiology, Duke University Medical Center, Durham, North Carolina.

Keri L. Fakata, PharmD, Research/Clinical Pharmacist, Pain Management/Palliative Care, Lifetree Pain Clinic; Clinical Instructor, College of Pharmacy, University of Utah, Salt Lake City, Utah; e-mail: <keri.fakata@hsc.utah.edu>.

Joseph F. Foss, MD, Director, Clinical Research, Adolor Corporation, Exton, Pennsylvania; e-mail: <jfoss@adolor.com>.

Tong J. Gan, MB, FRCA, FFARCSI, Associate Professor, Director, Clinical Research, Department of Anesthesiology, Duke University Medical Center, Durham, North Carolina; e-mail: <gan00001@ mc.duke.edu>.

Arthur G. Lipman, PharmD, FASHP, Professor, Department of Pharmacy Practice, College of Pharmacy, University of Utah, and Director, Clinical Pharmacology, University of Utah Hospitals and Clinics Pain Management Center, Salt Lake City, Utah; e-mail: <alipman@pharm.utah.edu>.

Sangeeta R. Mehendale, MD, PhD, Research Associate, Department of Anesthesia and Critical Care, Pritzker School of Medicine,

University of Chicago, Chicago, Illinois; e-mail: <smehendale@dacc.uchicago.edu>.

Jonathan Moss, MD, PhD, Professor, Department of Anesthesia and Critical Care, and Chairman, Institutional Review Board, University of Chicago, Chicago, Illinois; e-mail: <jm47@airway.uchicago.edu>.

Marco Pappagallo, MD, Director, Division of Chronic Pain, Department of Pain Medicine and Palliative Care, Beth Israel University Hospital, Manhattan Campus for the Albert Einstein College of Medicine, New York, New York; e-mail: <mpappaga@chpnet.org>.

William K. Schmidt, PhD, Vice President, Scientific Affairs, Adolor Corporation, Exton, Pennsylvania; e-mail: <wschmidt@adolor.com>.

Nigel P. Sykes, MA, FRCGP, Consultant Physician, Head of Medicine, St. Christopher's Hospice, Sydenham, London, United Kingdom; e-mail: <NIGELSYKES@doctors.org.uk>.

Ashok K. Tuteja, MD, MPH, Assistant Professor, Division of Gastroenterology, Department of Internal Medicine, University of Utah School of Medicine, Salt Lake City, Utah.

Gang Wei, MD, PhD, Director of Safety, Sigma-Tau Research, Inc., Gaithersburg, Maryland; e-mail: <gwei_5782@yahoo.com>.

Ysmael Yap, RPh, MD, Pain Fellow, Department of Pain Medicine and Palliative Care, Beth Israel Medical Center, Manhattan Campus for the Albert Einstein College of Medicine, New York, New York.

Preface

Opioid compounds, which are widely administered for a variety of medical indications, are associated with a number of side effects, especially opioid bowel dysfunction (OBD). Very often, OBD is so severe that physicians limit opioid use or dose, even when medically indicated. Although OBD is a significant clinical problem, it has received insufficient attention in the past by the medical community. The *Handbook of Opioid Bowel Syndrome* endeavors to rectify this neglect.

In the past two or three decades, progress has been made in understanding the mechanisms of action of opioids, and advances have been achieved in the management of OBD. These topics are discussed in depth in this book, which aims to provide complete, authoritative, and current information for physicians and other health care professionals. Currently, two peripheral opioid antagonists are being developed to potentially reverse OBD without affecting analgesia. These new compounds permit further understanding of the mechanisms of opioid effects and their therapeutic relevancy. Data obtained from the investigations of these novel compounds are also presented.

Many contributors have spent countless hours and *much energy* to update the information in this field. I sincerely appreciate their time and their wisdom shared in bringing this project to fruition. The work of this book was supported in part by National Institutes of Health grant R01 CA79042.

Introduction

Chun-Su Yuan
Marco Pappagallo

The opium poppy may have been used for several thousand years as a medicine to control diarrhea and relieve pain. In 1803, Friedrich Sertürner reported the isolation of a pure active alkaline substance from opium, and named it *morphine,* after Morpheus, the Greek god of dreams. Today, morphine and other opioids are widely used in different clinical settings, especially as analgesics to treat moderate to severe pain.

Although opioids are effective in managing acute and chronic pain, their most common and distressing adverse effect is bowel dysfunction. Opioid-induced bowel dysfunction (OBD), often described as constipation, is found in 90 percent of patients treated with opioids[1] and is a significant problem in 40 to 45 percent of patients with advanced cancer.[2,3] For chronic opioid substitute therapy, the literature has often concentrated on the effectiveness of the program, but opioid-induced constipation and the quantitative delay in gut transit time were reported.[4] OBD is characterized by a dry hard stool, straining during evacuation, incomplete evacuation, bloating, abdominal distension, cramping, nausea and vomiting, gastric reflux, and retention of gut contents.[5-7] After repeated use of opioids, tolerance develops for analgesia, euphoria, sedation, and respiratory suppression. However, tolerance does not appear to extend to the opioid effects on the gut.[4,8]

Complications associated with uncontrolled OBD include (1) fecal impaction and spurious diarrhea; (2) pseudo-obstruction of the bowel; and (3) interference with drug administration and absorption.[2,9] These consequences add to the discomfort of the patient and in many cases exacerbate pain and increase morbidity.[2,10] In palliative care (discussed in Chapter 5), the management of chronic OBD sometimes is more difficult than the control of pain. Despite aggressive use of laxatives, patients find that constipation persists. In severe cases, patients may choose to limit or discontinue opioid pain medications to reduce the pain and discomfort of OBD.[2,11] Persistent symptoms associated with OBD can have a negative impact on quality of life.[10,12] In addition, prolonged hospitalization in surgical patients with opioid-induced postoperative ileus (discussed in Chapters 7 and 8) increases health care costs.

Clinically, the severity of OBD may be influenced by opioid dose or formulation, titration schedule, previous opioid exposure, or polypharmacy.[10,13] Among the different opioid derivatives, OBD appears more pronounced with codeine than other agents.[7] In terms of formulation, transdermal opioids (e.g., fentanyl) are associated with significantly less constipation than the oral or parenteral formulations.[14]

Data from animal experiments also showed that the gastrointestinal tract was sensitive to opioids, even at low doses. The ratio of subcutaneous analgesic to constipating doses of morphine in the rat is approximately 4 to 1, i.e., four times more morphine is needed for analgesia than for gut effect.[15] In mice treated with oral doses of morphine, approximately 20 times less morphine was required to antagonize castor oil diarrhea than to produce analgesia.[16] Gut sensitivity to opioids is probably due to the poor penetration of morphine into the brain, which partly explains why OBD is a severe problem for patients treated with opioids.

Opioid receptors are widely distributed in the central nervous system and throughout the gastrointestinal tract. There are three primary opioid receptor subtypes: mu (μ), delta (δ), and kappa (κ). These receptors, stimulated by both endogenous (e.g., endorphin) and exogenous (e.g., morphine) agonists, are discussed in length in Chapters 1 and 2. The site of action of exogenous OBD, however, is somewhat controversial. In animals, morphine acts within the central nervous system to alter autonomic outflow to the gut.[17] But opioids have also been shown to change intestinal motility by a direct effect on the bowel. Morphine inhibits gastric transit primarily from direct action on the gut at opioid sites, with little contribution from a centrally elicited effect.[18] Loperamide, an opioid receptor agonist with limited ability to access the central nervous system, is used to treat diarrhea, suggesting that direct, local action on the gut by opioids causes constipation in humans. Using a muscle strip preparation of human small intestine, we demonstrated that morphine-induced inhibition of contraction is blocked by opioid antagonists.[19] In addition, contraction in the muscle strip was up to 27 percent greater with opioid antagonists than at control levels, suggesting inhibitory modulation in the gut by endogenous opioids in humans.

The gastrointestinal effects of morphine are mediated primarily by μ receptors in the bowel.[20,21] By inhibiting gastric emptying and reducing propulsive peristalsis of the intestine, morphine decreases the rate of intestinal transit. Reduction in gut secretion and increases in intestinal fluid absorption also contribute to the constipating effect. Opioids also may act on the gut indirectly through tonic gut spasms after inhibition of nitric oxide generation. This effect was shown in animals when a nitric oxide precusor reversed morphine-induced changes in gut motility.[22,23] It appears that the mechanisms for OBD are multifactorial, encompassing both the opioid and nonopioid neuromodulatory systems.

In this monograph, we present basic concepts in OBD and discuss its management in several clinical settings. In addition, two selective peripheral opioid antagonists, methylnaltrexone and alvimopan, currently under clinical investigation, are introduced in Chapters 10 and 11. These novel peripheral opioid antagonists have the potential not only to prevent or treat OBD but also to provide us with an opportunity to elucidate the mechanism of actions of the peripheral effects of opioids in humans.

NOTES

1. Twycross RG, Lack SA. *Symptom control in far advanced cancer: Pain relief.* London: Pitman; 1983.

2. Walsh TD. Oral morphine in chronic cancer pain. *Pain* 1984;18:1-11.

3. Glare P, Lickiss JN. Unrecognized constipation in patients with advanced cancer: A recipe for therapeutic disaster. *J Pain Symptom Manage* 1992;7:369-371.

4. Yuan CS, Foss JF, Moss J, Roizen MF. Gut motility and transit changes in patients receiving long-term methadone maintenance. *J Clin Pharmacol* 1998;38:931-935.

5. Livingston EH, Passaro EP Jr. Postoperative ileus. *Dig Dis Sci* 1990;35:121-132.

6. Pappagallo M. Incidence, prevalence, and management of opioid bowel dysfunction. *Am J Surg* 2001;182(5A Suppl):11S-18S.

7. Kurz A, Sessler DI. Opioid-induced bowel dysfunction: Pathophysiology and potential new therapies. *Drugs* 2003;63:649-671.

8. Walsh TD. Prevention of opioid side effects. *J Pain Symptom Manage* 1990;5:362-367.

9. Mercadante S, Fulfaro F, Casuccio A. The impact of home palliative care on symptoms in advanced cancer patients. *Support Care Cancer* 2000;8:307-310.

10. Klepstad P, Kaasa S, Skauge M, Borchgrevink PC. Pain intensity and side effects during titration of morphine to cancer patients using a fixed schedule dose escalation. *Acta Anaesthesiol Scand* 2000;44:656-664.

11. Whitecar PS, Jonas AP, Clasen ME. Managing pain in the dying patient. *Am Fam Physician* 2000;61:755-764.

12. Fallon MT, Hanks GW. Morphine, constipation, and performance status in advanced cancer patients. *Palliat Med* 1999;13:159-160.

13. Sykes NP. The relationship between opioid use and laxative use in terminally ill cancer patients. *Palliat Med* 1998;12:375-382.

14. Ahmedzai S, Brooks D. Transdermal fentanyl versus sustained-release oral morphine in cancer pain: Preference, efficacy, and quality of life. The TTS-Fentanyl Comparative Trial Group. *J Pain Symptom Manage* 1997;13:254-261.

15. Green AF. Comparative effects of analgesics on pain threshold, respiratory frequency and gastrointestinal propulsion. *Br J Pharmacol* 1959;14:26-34.

16. Niemegeers C, Lenaerts F, Awouters F. Preclinical animal studies of modern antidiarrheal: in vivo pharmacology. In Van Bever W, Lal H (eds.), *Synthetic antidiarrheal drugs: Synthesis-preclinical and clinical pharmacology.* New York: Marcel Dekker; 1976:65-114.

17. Galligan JJ, Burks TF. Centrally mediated inhibition of small intestinal transit and motility by morphine in the rat. *J Pharmacol Exp Ther* 1983;226:356-361.

18. Manara L, Bianchi G, Ferretti P, Tavani A. Inhibition of gastrointestinal transit by morphine in rats results primarily from direct drug action on gut opioid sites. *J Pharmacol Exp Ther* 1986;237:945-949.

19. Yuan CS, Foss JF, Moss J. Effects of methylnaltrexone on morphine-induced inhibition of contraction in isolated guinea-pig ileum and human intestine. *Eur J Pharmacol* 1995;276:107-111.

20. De Luca A, Coupar IM. Insights into opioid action in the intestinal tract. *Pharmacol Ther* 1996;69:103-115.

21. Reisine T, Pasternak G. Opioid analgesics and antagonists. In Hardman JG, Gilman AG, Limbird LE (eds.), *Goodman & Gilman's: The pharmacological basis of therapeutics,* 9th ed. New York: McGraw-Hill; 1996:521-555.

22. Calignano A, Moncada S, Di Rosa M. Endogenous nitric oxide modulates morphine-induced constipation. *Biochem Biophys Res Commun* 1991;181:889-893.

23. Karan RS, Kumar R, Pandhi P. Effect of acute and chronic administration of L-arginine on morphine induced inhibition of gastrointestinal motility. *Indian J Physiol Pharmacol* 2000;44:345-349.

SECTION I:
BASIC CONCEPTS IN OPIOID
BOWEL DYSFUNCTION

Chapter 1

Gastrointestinal Opioid Physiology and Pharmacology

Keri L. Fakata
Arthur G. Lipman

Opioids inhibit gastrointestinal (GI) motility, especially by binding at and activating (acting as agonists at) mu (μ) opioid receptors in the intestinal tract. The major mechanism for the effect of these drugs on bowel function is believed to be activation of these receptors in the colon. The resulting inhibition of peristalsis can produce opioid-induced constipation. This chapter briefly reviews the physiology and pharmacology associated with the binding of opioids to opioid receptors in the GI tract. It provides a brief overview of normal GI motility and what occurs when opioids bind to the receptors, interrupting bowel homeostasis.

GASTROINTESTINAL PHYSIOLOGY

Normal Gastrointestinal Motility

Normal GI motility results from coordinated smooth muscle contractions that originate in myocytes and are produced by two patterns of electrical activity: slow wave and spike potentials. On the cellular level, myocytes differ in the stomach and small intestine from those found in the colon. The myocytes in the stomach and small intestine contain gap junctions that allow the current to easily pass from one cell to the next allowing the stomach and the small intestines to function as a unit, resulting in coordinated contractions. Because the myocytes in the colon do not contain gap junctions, they do not act as a unit, and extrinsic input is required to coordinate smooth muscle cell activity.[1] In the electrically coupled myocytes of the stomach and small intestine, small (5 to 15 millivolts [mV]) fluctuations in membrane potential, called slow waves, are observed. The slow waves occur 10 to 20 times per minute in the small intestine and 3 to 8 times per minute in the stomach and large intestine.[2] The slow waves are not action potentials; they do not elicit contractions. Rather, they are rolling changes in the resting membrane potential.

The second type of electrical activity is the spike wave, an action potential that occurs at the crest of the slow wave which elicits contractions in response to local neurotransmitter release. This release, in turn, is a response to distention by a food bolus. The food bolus occurs after feeding, producing a fed state with constant ungrouped, low varying amplitude contractions, which are dependent upon the volume and chemical contents of the ingested food.[2] During periods of fasting and between meals, a pattern of bowel activity termed the migrating motor complex (MMC) propels GI contents distally.[3] The MMC is initiated every one to two hours, and there are four phases to the complex. Phase I consists of oscillating slow wave, smooth muscle action potentials with intermittent spike wave potentials that initiate phase II. Phase III is initiated when the frequency of the contractions increase to about 3 per minute in the stomach and 11 per minute in the duodenum. The contractions migrate in an orderly manner, beginning in the stomach and ending at the ileum. Bowel quiescence signifies phase IV of the MMC. The MMC is important because it is the only stimulatory process in the GI tract for patients who have not eaten due to illness or procedures, e.g., patients who cannot eat due to surgery.[3]

Functional Movements of the GI Tract

Myocytes, the cells that constitute the circular and longitudinal muscle layers in the GI tract, propel the GI contents distally. The two types of movements of these muscles propel and mix the intralumenal material. Stretching of the gut wall by a food bolus elicits the propulsive movement called peristalsis; coordinated, bandlike contractions of the circular muscles proximal to the bolus and relaxation of the muscles distal to the bolus move the food down the GI tract. The mixing motion is initiated in the small intestine and proximal colon. This motion facilitates absorption of nutrients and fluids by exposing maximum surface area of the material to the intestinal mucosa. Both types of movements are controlled by the enteric nervous system with input from the autonomic nervous system.[1,4]

Enteric Nervous System

The enteric nervous system (ENS) has been called "the body's second brain."[5] Bayliss and Starling demonstrated by the extrinsic denervation of canine intestines that gut contains a nervous system of its own. Trendelenburg later supported this finding of preserved peristaltic reflexes in isolated guinea pig gut.[5] The ENS consists of two major ganglionic plexi: the myenteric plexus and the submucosal plexus,[5] as shown in Figure 1.1. The enteric plexi contain sensory neurons, motor neurons, and interneurons. Sensory neurons receive messages from sensory receptors in the mucosa that respond to mechanical, thermal, osmotic, and chemical stimuli. Motor neurons control GI motility, secretion, and absorption by acting directly upon

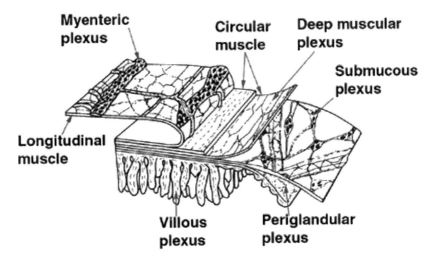

FIGURE 1.1. The enteric nervous system (www.open.ac.uk/science/biosci/research/saffrey/Fig2.gif). *Source:* Copyright The Open University. Originally published in Furness, JB and Costa, M. Types of nerves in the enteric nervous system. *Neuroscience* 1980;5(1):1-20.

effector cells, such as those found in smooth muscle and secretory cells. The interneurons compile information from the sensory neurons and link it to the motor neurons.[6] The myenteric plexus lies between the circular and longitudinal muscles of the muscularis externa. This plexus contains a large number of neurons, a number that rivals the quantity of cells found in the CNS. This plexus controls GI motor activity and mediates secretory output of such organs as the pancreas and gallbladder. The submucosal plexus lies within the GI submucosa and contains sensory neurons that communicate with the myenteric plexus and motor neurons, which control local secretory and absorptive activities within the gut lumen.[6]

Local Enteric Nervous System Factors

Several neurotransmitters that are also found in the CNS are released from the enteric neurons. Acetylcholine, the major neurotransmitter produced by enteric neurons, stimulates GI motility. Several other factors either stimulate or inhibit GI motility; their effects are listed in Table 1.1.[3,7]

Autonomic Control

The parasympathetic and sympathetic branches of the autonomic nervous system innervate the enteric plexi. Parasympathetic input is delivered by the vagus nerve that innervates the esophagus, stomach, and the proximal half of the large intestine. The distal colon receives parasympathetic input from the pelvic nerves. Parasympathetic activity is additive to ENS activity, increasing GI motor activity. Sympathetic (splanchnic) neural impulses inhibit the release of acetylcholine from neurons in the myenteric plexus.[3] The release of norepinephrine by the sympathetic nerve endings inhibits the ENS and decreases GI motor activity.[1]

Central Nervous System

Although the ENS can function independently, normal GI function requires an intact autonomic (parasympathetic and sympathetic) nervous system that communicates between the gut and the brain. If the

TABLE 1.1. Effects of neurotransmitters, local factors, and hormones on GI motility.

Factors	Mechanisms	
	Stimulatory	**Inhibitory**
Acetylcholine	✓	
Norepinephrine		✓
Dopamine	✓	
Serotonin	✓	✓
Vasoactive intestinal peptide (VIP)		✓
Substance P (SP)	✓	✓
Nitric oxide		✓
Gastrin	✓	
Cholecystokinin (CCK)	✓	
Motilin	✓	
Prostaglandins	✓	
Bradykinins	✓	
Bombesin	✓	
Neurotensin	✓	
Somatostatin		✓
Glucagon		✓
Gastric inhibitory peptide		✓
Calcitonin gene-related peptide		✓
Corticotropin releasing factor		✓
Endogenous opioids		✓

Sources: Luckey A, Livingston E, Tache Y. Mechanisms and treatment of postoperative ileus. *Arch Surg* 2003;138:206-214; Kromer W. Endogenous and exogenous opioids in the control of gastrointestinal motility and secretion. *Pharmacol Rev* 1988;40:121-162; Kromer W. The current status of opioid research on gastrointestinal motility. *Life Sci* 1989;44:579-589; De Luca A, Coupar IM. Insights into opioid action in the intestinal tract. *Pharmacol Ther* 1996;69:103-115.

gut signals the brain that a toxic substance has been ingested, the brain initiates the vomiting reflex. The brain receives olfactory and visual signals related to feeding/food that result in efferent stimulation of the gut to release digestive enzymes.[5]

OPIOID EFFECTS
ON THE GASTROINTESTINAL SYSTEM

Opioids are known to slow gastrointestinal transit. The clinical effect of constipation due to opioids is well-known but has not been quantified. Recent advances have characterized the effects of opioids on gut function, and research in this area is ongoing. Areas of research include the identification and location of opioid receptors in the gastrointestinal tract, the actions of endogenous and exogenous opioids at the receptor site, and the effects of local factors that affect GI motility.

Opioid Receptors

Six types of opioid receptors have been identified and three of these are known to have clinically important effects in humans. These are classified as mu (μ), delta (δ), and kappa (κ) receptors, all of which have subtypes. Both exogenous and endogenous opioid compounds can activate the opioid receptors. The opioid receptors belong to the G protein couple receptor family. When stimulated, the opioid receptor on the cellular level decreases calcium influx resulting in (1) a decrease of presynaptic neurotransmitter release, (2) an increase of potassium influx resulting in hypopolarization of postsynaptic neurons, and (3) local GABAergic transmission.[8] Most of what is known about the opioid receptors is derived from clinical observation in humans and animal studies. Physiological roles of these three opioid receptor types are listed in Table 1.2.[8] Three types of endogenous opioid peptides are located in the CNS and periphery: enkephalins, endorphins, and dynorphins. The endorphins have the greatest affinity for the μ receptor, the enkephalins are endogenous ligands for the δ receptor, and dynorphins have greatest affinity for the κ receptor. These endogenous opioid peptides are found in high concentrations within areas of the brain responsible for pain perception, modulation of affective behavior, motor control, regulation of the autonomic nervous system, and neuroendocrine function. Opioid peptides found in the periphery may have such roles as neuroimmune modulation and normal bowel motility. Gastrointestinal effects of endogenous opioid peptides are further discussed in the Chapter 2, and those of exogenous opioids are discussed later in this chapter.

TABLE 1.2. Physiological profile of three classic opioid receptors.

Function	Opioid receptor	Action
Analgesia	μ, κ, δ	Pain relief
Respiratory	μ, κ, δ	Depression of function
Cough	μ?	Depression
Immune function	μ	Increase/decrease
Skin	μ	Itching
Gastrointestinal tract	μ, κ, . . . δ?	Decrease motility
Pupil effect	μ, κ	Miosis
Psychoactivity	κ	Increase
Feeding	μ, κ, δ	Increase
Sedation	μ, κ	Increase
Urinary retention	μ, κ	Decrease/increase
Hormone regulation	μ,κ	Variable effects
Neurotransmitter release	μ, κ, δ	Variable effects

Sources: Kurz A, Sessler DI. Opioid-induced bowel dysfunction: Pathophysiology and potential new therapies. *Drugs* 2003;63:649-671; Reisine T, Paternak G. Opioid analgesic and antagonists. In Hardman JG, Limbird LE, Gilman AG (eds.), *Goodman & Gilman's The pharmacological basis of therapeutics.* New York: McGraw-Hill, 1996:521-555.

All three types of opioid receptors have been isolated in the GI tracts of several animal species.[7] The effects of opioids on the bowel are primarily mediated by μ receptors; the roles of δ and κ receptors are less clear.[9,10] Available opioids do not discriminate between $μ_1$ and $μ_2$ receptor subtypes. When an opioid is administered systemically, $μ_1$ receptor agonist effects produce supraspinal analgesia, and $μ_2$ receptor activation causes several effects, including respiratory depression and constipation.

Interspecies variability is observed in the distribution of opioid receptors in the GI tract.[9] Most in vitro animal studies have been performed using guinea pig ileum. Radiolabeled ligand binding studies demonstrate that both μ and κ receptors are located on the plasma membrane of the cholinergic nerve terminals of the longitudinal muscle myenteric plexus and inhibit the release of acetylcholine.[11] Inhibition of acetylcholine slows GI motility and dries secretions, contributing to opioid-induced constipation. Inhibitory action of opioids on peristalsis has been demonstrated in vitro in guinea pigs, rat, cats, and rabbits, whereas excitatory effects have occurred in dogs and cats.[7,9] Variability in the opioid effects on gut motility depends not only on species but also on section of the gastrointestinal tract (small versus large intestine), the particular segment within a part (e.g., proximal versus distal colon), the dose of peptides, the technique used to measure gastrointestinal motility, and the feeding state of the animal, and is caused by difference in distribution of opioid receptor subtypes in the gut.[12-14] It has therefore been difficult to compare and contrast variability among species due to the various confounding factors and inconsistent study conditions.[9,10]

Opioid receptors are found both in the central nervous system and the periphery. It is difficult to define the location and specific mechanism of opioid effects on the GI tract. It is not clear whether the effects are central, peripheral, or a combination of the two.

Central Opioid Effects on GI Motility

Evidence for a central effect of opioids on GI motility comes from several animal studies in which morphine, other exogenous opioids, or endogenous opioid peptides were injected directly into areas of the brain. Slowed GI transit time was seen in several animals. Initial postulations regarding CNS effects from opioids that impact GI motility include μ receptor activation, effects on vagal pathways that link the brain and the enteric nervous system, and possible release of an unknown humoral substance released from the brain.[10] The μ receptors are involved in the inhibition of gastrointestinal function at the central and spinal level.[15-17] The central and spinal effects of κ and δ agonists on slowing gastrointestinal transit appear to be unclear.[16-19]

Several arguments can be made against an entirely central cause of opioid-induced constipation. The distribution and metabolism characteristics of an opioid given systemically must be considered when it is being delivered locally. The animal results are variable between species. Small local doses of opioid were required to decrease GI transit in the mouse, whereas large local doses were required in the rat, compared to the systemic doses needed to achieve the opioid effect on the bowel.[10] Clinical experience in humans with central administration opioids (e.g., intrathecal morphine), does not cause constipation because little morphine is available peripherally. Studies done in the rat model resemble that the clinical experience of humans.[10] In addition, the development of methylnaltrexone, a novel peripheral opioid antagonist that is discussed later in this chapter (also in Chapter 10) is more consistent with a peripheral mechanism for opioid-induced constipation. The development of peripheral, selective opioid agonists and antagonists has proven beneficial in determining the peripheral and central effects of opioids on the GI tract.

Peripheral Opioid Effects on GI Motility

The presence of opioid receptors in the GI tract of humans and other species suggests peripheral opioid action. Local administration of morphine to rat intestines in vivo slowed intestinal propulsion.[20] The comparison of intraperitoneal and intravenous morphine in the rat model demonstrated greater intestinal morphine concentration with the local injection which correlated with constipation.[20] Observations in humans and other species show that significantly less opioids are needed to induce constipation than is required for analgesia.[10,21,22] Thus, it would be expected that similar small doses of opioid antagonist would be required to reverse constipation. Interestingly, tolerance does not occur with constipation as it does for other effects of opioids, such as sedation and respiratory depression.[23]

Peripheral Opioid Receptor Stimulation

Both the enteric and the autonomic nervous system are known to release acetylcholine, which increases GI motility. Cherubini and North evaluated the ionic mechanisms for the inhibition of release of acetylcholine in cell somata of the guinea pig myenteric neuron after stimulation by several different opioid preparations. The results suggest that acetylcholine release is inhibited by different mechanisms dependent upon the class of receptors.[24] Activation of μ receptors increases potassium conductance in the cell that may shorten the presynaptic action potential, therefore decreasing neurotransmitter release. Nishiwaki et al. demonstrated that endogenous opioids might play a role in acetylcholine release via the μ receptor when muscarinic autoinhibition is altered.[25] Stimulation of κ receptors reduces calcium entry into the cell through voltage-regulated channels. The stimulated κ receptor inhibits the release of acetylcholine, regardless of muscarinic activity in the electric-field-stimulated guinea pig ileum.[25] The δ receptor does not appear to have a role in acetylcholine release in the guinea pig ileum.[24] This study demonstrates different ionic mechanisms of opioid-mediated inhibition of acetylcholine release.

Antisecretory Effect of Opioids

Stimulation of the enteric μ receptors by opioids increases fluid absorption from the intestines. Initially, the antidiarrheal properties of opioids were thought to originate from stimulation of the sympathetic branch of the nervous system. The assumption was that decreased GI motility prolongs GI transit time, increasing time for absorption of fluids and electrolytes. However, the antidiarrheal mechanism of opioids is far more complex. The human GI system is contributing 9 L/day of the approximate 40 L of fluid in the human body. This fluid comes from the recommended daily intake of 2 L of water and secretions produced by the salivary glands, stomach, and pancreas.[13] Opioids have an effect on the release of neurotransmitter and hormones that affects the release of secretion from organs. The development of peripherally acting μ agonists for the treatment of traveler's diarrhea answered many questions about opioid antisecretory properties. These peripherally acting antidiarrheal agents are commercially available as diphenoxylate (Lomotil) and loperamide (Imodium A-D). The peripheral mechanism of morphine and diphenoxylate is thought to act on μ receptors on the myenteric plexus, submucosa, villus core, and crypt regions.[13] Serotonin released from the myenteric plexus stimulates release of norepinephrine, which has sympathomimetic effects that decrease secretions. The mechanism of action of loperamide differs; it does not require norepinephrine for its antisecretory action.[13]

Opioids, especially endogenous opioid ligands, may interact with local mediators to affect secretion. Effects of local mediators on the GI tract are listed in Table 1.1. Several local factors are thought to coexist with endogenous opioids in the ENS. They may also exist in separate neurons and provide positive and negative feedback mechanisms to control normal bowel function. Exogenous opioids may counteract this homeostasis. In vitro animal studies indicate that vasoactive inhibitory polypeptide (VIP) is a nonadrenergic inhibitory neurotransmitter that affects GI motility. Opioids may inhibit VIP release. Cholecystokinin (CCK) favors release of both endogenous opioids and substance P (SP). In turn, endogenous opioids inhibit the release of excitatory SP through negative feedback.[7,9,13] These findings and speculations indicate the need for further research on the interactions of endogenous and exogenous opioids with GI neurotransmitters and neuromodulators. Since endogenous opioids may play a role in certain gastrointestinal diseases, endogenous opioid peptides will be further discussed in Chapter 2, which focuses on the pathophysiology of opioid-induced bowel dysfunction.

Summary

Figure 1.2 illustrates the effects of opioids on the enteric nervous system. Clinical observations and both animal and human studies have led to generalizations about the effects of opioids on GI function. Table 1.3 summarizes these effects.

EXOGENOUS OPIOID EFFECTS ON THE GASTROINTESTINAL SYSTEM

Opioid Agonists

Several opioid analgesics are commercially available. Opioids analgesics combined with nonopioid analgesics (e.g., acetaminophen or ibuprofen) are commonly used to treat moderate to moderately severe pain. These combined formulations have a dose ceiling that is due not to the opioid ingredient but to the acetaminophen and ibuprofen. The dose should be titrated to achieve maximum analgesia and minimum side effects. Tolerance develops quickly to CNS effects such sedation, respiratory depression, nausea, and vomiting. Tolerance is slow to develop, if at all, for peripheral side effects such as constipation and urinary retention. Physical dependence develops rapidly; this should not be confused with addiction. Physical dependence is characterized by a withdrawal phenomenon if the opioid is stopped too rapidly or an antagonist is administered. Discontinuation of an opioid

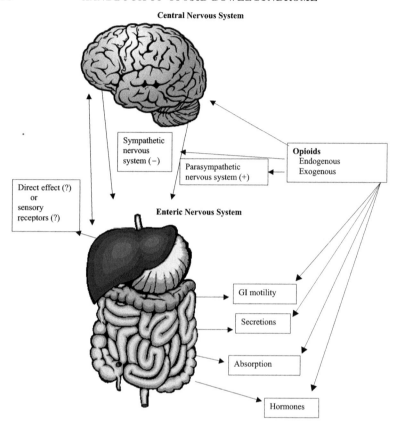

FIGURE 1.2. Effects of opioids on the enteric and central nervous systems. *Sources:* Kurz A, Sessler DI. Opioid-induced bowel dysfunction: Pathophysiology and potential new therapies. *Drugs* 2003;63:649-671; Kromer W. Endogenous and exogenous opioids in the control of gastrointestinal motility and secretion. *Pharmacol Rev* 1988;40:121-162; Manara L, Bianchetti A. The central and peripheral influences of opioids on gastrointestinal propulsion. *Annu Rev Pharmacol Toxicol* 1985;25:249-273; De Luca A, Coupar IM. Insights into opioid action in the intestinal tract. *Pharmacol Ther* 1996;69:103-115.

should be accomplished with a dose taper over five to ten days to avoid effects such as diarrhea, nausea, flulike symptoms, tremor, and anxiety.[26]

When compared to the analgesic efficacy of morphine, no one opioid stands out above the other. Opioid analgesics differ in analgesic potency, pharmacokinetics, and dosage forms for a range of routes

TABLE 1.3. Accepted opioid effects on GI motility.

Area of gastrointestinal tract	Effect
Stomach	Delayed gastric emptying
	Increased antral tone in proximal duodenum
Small intestine	Inhibited intestinal transit (biphasic)
	Stimulatory via activation of MMC phase III
	Followed by atony
Colon	Increased tone and amplitude of nonpropulsive contractions
	Decreased propulsive waves in the colon
Gastrointestinal sphincters	Increased pressure
	Decreased relaxation
Net effect	Decreased in GI motility

Sources: Kurz A, Sessler DI. Opioid-induced bowel dysfunction: Pathophysiology and potential new therapies. *Drugs* 2003;63:649-671; Reisine T, Paternak G. Opioid analgesic and antagonists. In Hardman JG, Limbird LE, Gilman AG (eds.), *Goodman & Gilman's The pharmacological basis of therapeutics.* New York: McGraw-Hill, 1996:521-555.

of administration. These differences are listed in Table 1.4. There can also be variability in how an individual may respond to a single opioid preparation. For example, one patient may have significant nausea and vomiting with morphine. However, when changed to another opioid analgesic such as oxycodone, these side effects may diminish. The same scenario is also true for the analgesic properties in the individual. One patient may achieve better pain control with one opioid than another. Recent advances in opioid pharmacology have elucidated genetic polymorphisms in both murine and human μ receptor genes that are thought to be partially responsible for these interindividual differences.[27] These genetic polymorphisms may alter how the receptor is expressed on the cell surface and physiologic responses when the receptor is stimulated or blocked, for example, in the bowel. Rotation of opioids should be considered when a patient is experiencing problematic side effects or is not obtaining adequate analgesia despite multiple dose escalations.[28]

TABLE 1.4. Comparison of commercially available opioids.

Drug	Administration	Equianalgesic oral dosing (mg)	Equianalgesic parenteral dosing (mg)	Equianalgesic dosing interval (hours)	Half-life (hours)	Active metabolites	Precaution/ comments
Morphine sulfate (MS Contin, Oramorph SR, Kadian, AVINZA, MSIR)	PO, IV, SQ, IM, SL, RT, IT, EP	15 SR 30 IR	5 5	8-12 4-6	2-3.5	M-6-G M-3-G	M-6-G accumulation in renal insufficency
Codeine	PO, IV	65	30	4-6	3	Morphine M-6-G M-3-G	Do not exceed 65-100 mg, increase in side effects, pruritus, nausea, constipation
Methadone (Dolophine)	PO, IV, SQ	10	5	6-8	13-50	None known	Incomplete cross tolerance between morphine makes equianalgesic dosing difficult. Careful titration-accumulation occurs in first 5-10 days.
Levorphanol (Levo-Dromoran)	PO, IV	2	1	6-8	12-16	None known	Same as Methadone
Hydromorphone (Dilaudid)	PO, IV, SQ, IT, EP	2-4	1-2	4	2-3	M-6-G M-3-G	May use in patients with allergy to morphine. Safest opioid in patients with renal and liver failure.

Oxycodone (OxyContin, Oxy IR, Percocet, Percodan, Roxicodone, Roxicet)	PO	10	N/A	8-12 SR 4-6 IR	2-3	Oxymorphone	Dose ceiling for combination products with acetaminophen ≤4,000 mg of acetaminophen/day
Merperidine (Demerol)	IV, IM, PO	150	50-75	2.5-3.5		Normer-peridine	Active metabolite half-life 13-21 hr, accumulation occurs in healthy individuals, neurotoxicity Limit use to ≤ 2 days
Hydrocodone (various)	PO combination with APAP or Ibuprophen	See comments	See comments	See comments	See comments	See comments	Kenetics not well described. Many clinicians consider it equivalent to oxycodone.
Fentanyl (Duragesic, Actiq)	Transdermal transmucosal IV	25 µg/72 hours 200 µg to 60 µg morphine/day	25 µg/72 hours	72 hours (48 in some patients)[a]	17 hours 7 hours	N/A	Not for use in opioid-naive patients.

aDue to interpatient variability in skin permeability and clearance of fentanyl, some patients may require an interval of every 48 hours. It is recommended that a dosage increase be tried before increasing the interval. *Sources:* Adapted from American Pain Society. *Principles of analgesic use in the treatment of acute pain and chronic cancer pain,* 5th ed. Glenview, IL: American Pain Society; 2003; Hardman JG, Limbird LE, Gilman AG (eds.), *Goodman & Gilman's The pharmacological basis of therapeutics.* New York: McGraw-Hill, 1996:521-555; Inturrisi CE. Clinical pharmacology of opioids for pain. *Clin J Pain* 2002;18:S3-S13.

21

Agonist-Antagonist and Partial-Agonist Analgesics

These two classes of opioid analgesics are thought to have less abuse potential; however, their utilization is limited due to side effects, an analgesic dose ceiling, and the routes by which they can be administered. Because of the ceiling effect, it is more difficult to produce respiratory depression with these agents. It is also difficult to escalate the dose to achieve adequate pain control due to an increase in psychotomimetic effect, e.g., pentazocine. These agents may precipitate withdrawal in a patient tolerant to µ agonist opioid analgesics due to displacement of the latter from the µ receptors.[28] A summary of the mixed agonist-antagonist and the one available partial-agonist opioid analgesic is listed in Table 1.5.

Do Different Opioids Have Varying Effects
on the Gastrointestinal System?

An early rat study evaluated the effects of five opioid agonists (morphine, methadone, diamorphine [heroin], etorphine, and meperidine [pethidine]) on gastrointestinal transit using the charcoal meal test. Etorphine and meperidine were antagonized by intracereboventricular administration of naloxone and thought to have a primary central effect on the bowel. Morphine was fully antagonized by intraperitoneal N-methyl-naloxone and thought to act primarily in the periphery. Diamorphine and methadone were only partially antagonized by both types of antagonist administration.[29]

Some studies with transdermal fentanyl have claimed less constipation and laxative use compared to morphine. A long-term observation study of fentanyl in 73 cancer patients reported low incidence of constipation. The results were reported in number per treatment month and 72 percent of patient months were free of constipation.[30] This is thought to be due to the lipophilicity of fentanyl making it less available to the periphery compared to morphine. Clinically, all opioids cause constipation; the extent of constipation and tolerability is patient variable. If constipation cannot be managed, opioid rotation may be beneficial.

TABLE 1.5. Comparison of partial and mixed agonist-antagonist opioids.

Drug	Approximate equianalgesic oral dose (mg)	Approximate equianalgesic parenteral dose (mg)	Approximate onset PO, parenteral (min)	Equianalgesic dosing inverval (hours)	Comments
Buprenorphine (Buprenex)	Not available	0.1-0.2	N/A, 25	6-8	Partial agonist
Butorphanol (Stadol, Stadol NS)	Not available	1	N/A, 20	3-4	Available as a nasal spray
Nalbuphine (Nubain)	Not available	5	N/A, 20	3-6	
Pentazocine (Talwin Nx)	75	30	20, 15	3-6	Hallucinations

Source: Adapted from Choi YS, Billings JA. Opioid antagonists: A review of their role in palliative care, focusing on use in opioid-related constipation. J Pain Symptom Manage 2002;24:71-90.

Opioid Antagonists

Opioid antagonists are synthetic derivatives of morphine or oxymorphine that compete with endogenous and exogenous opioids for the opioid receptors.[31] They are most commonly administered to counteract opioid toxicity, such as respiratory depression. These agents have also been used and studied to treat intolerable side effects such as pruritus, constipation, nausea, and vomiting; however, their use is often avoided due to concern about reversing analgesia and precipitating withdrawal. Studies of naloxone for the treatment of opioid-induced constipation will be addressed in Chapter 6. Currently three opioid antagonists are available on the market. A summary of their pharmacokinetics is shown in Table 1.6.[31] Naloxone (Narcan) is available only as an injection, and is Food and Drug Administration (FDA) approved for the treatment of opioid overdose, postoperative opioid depression, and septic shock. Naltrexone (ReVia) is a long-acting oral dosage form that is FDA approved for the treatment of alchohol dependence and opioid addiction. Nalmefene HCl (Revex) is a longer-acting parenteral used to treat opioid overdose and postoperative opioid depression. It may be required for the reversal of opioid-induced respiratory depression caused by the pharmacologically longer-acting opioids agonists, such as methadone. Peripheral opioid antagonists such as methylnaltrexone and alvimopan are currently being investigated for the treatment of opioid-induced side effects with a focus on opioid-induced constipation. Methylnaltrexone is a peripheral pure μ antagonist, a quaternary derivative of naltrexone with a methyl group at the amine. This affords the molecule greater polarity and lower lipid solubility, which prevents the molecules from crossing the blood-brain barrier. Methylnaltrexone is glucuronidated by the liver and about half is excreted unchanged in the urine. Early studies in rodents found that methylnaltrexone could be demethylated to naltrexone in murine species. However, humans lack this demethylating enzyme and therefore cannot metabolize it into naltrexone.[32] Alvimopan is a potent peripheral μ antagonist that has lower affinity for δ and κ receptors. It is a small synthetic zwitterionic piperidine molecule with a high molecular weight. It is poorly absorbed from the gastrointestinal tract with a reported bioavailibility of 0.03 percent after administration in dogs and rabbits.[33] After intravenous administration alvimopan was found throughout the body of

TABLE 1.6. Pharmacokinetics of opioid antagonists available in the United States.

	Administration/onset	Absorption	Distribution	Metabolism	Elimination
Naloxone (Narcan)	Endotracehal, IM Onset 2-5 min IV Onset 2 min Duration 20-60 min	Oral = rapidly inactivated	VDss 180-210	Rapid by glucuronidation in the liver Half-life 1-1.5 h	Urine metabolites
Naltrexone (ReVia)	PO Onset 60 min Duration 24-72 h	Complete	VDss 191/kg Protein binding 21%	Extensive first pass Several metabolites 6-β-naltrexol: 13 h Half-life: 10 h Terminal Half-life 96 h	Metabolites and unchanged drug in urine
Nalmefene (Revex)	IM Onset 15 min SC Onset 15 min IV Onset 2-5 min Duration 2-8 h	100% IM, SC	VDss 8.61/kg Protein binding 45%	Glucuronidation by the liver Half-life: 8.5-10.8 h	Renal <8% Feces 17% Bile—small

Sources: Adapted from Schmidt WK. Alvimopan (ADL 8-2698) is a novel peripheral opioid antagonist. *Am J Surg* 2001;182:27S-38S; Choi YS, Billings JA. Opioid antagonists: A review of their role in palliative care, focusing on use in opioid-related constipation. *J Pain Symptom Manage* 2002;24:71-90.

the rat except for the brain and spinal cord. These agents will be discussed in greater detail in future chapters.

Summary

Opioids are a mainstay in the treatment of moderate to severe pain. They are associated with many side effects that may limit dose escalation needed to effectively treat pain. Constipation is one of the common side effects that may affect how adequately pain is treated. The mechanism of opioid-induced constipation is complex with multiple interactions among the enteric nervous system, local mediators, and the central nervous system. The development of peripheral opioid antagonists has provided not only better understanding of these mechanisms but also what appears to be a safe and effective treatment for opioid-induced constipation without concern for reversal of analgesia.

I have finally come to the konklusin that a good set of bowels iz worth more to a man than enny quantity of brains.

Josh Billings, aka Henry Wheeler Shaw, 1818-1885 an American writer known for his intentional misspellings[6]

NOTES

1. Kurz A, Sessler DI. Opioid-induced bowel dysfunction: Pathophysiology and potential new therapies. *Drugs* 2003;63:649-671.

2. Bowen R. Electrophysiology of the gastrointestinal smooth muscle (November 23, 1996). Available at <http://arbl.cymbs.colostate.edu/hbooks/pathphs/digestion/basics/slowwaves.htm>.

3. Luckey A, Livingston E, Tache Y. Mechanisms and treatment of postoperative ileus. *Arch Surg* 2003;138:206-214.

4. Bowen R. Gastrointestinal motility and smooth muscle (July 8, 2002). Available at <http://arbl.cymbs.colostate.edu/hbooks/pathphys/digestion/basics/gi_motility.html>.

5. Gershon M. The enteric nervous system: A second brain. Available at <http://www.hospitalpract.com/issues/1999/07/gershon.htm>.

6. Bowen R. The enteric nervous system (1998). Available at <http://arbl.cymbs.colostate.edu/hbooks/pathphys/digestion/basics/gi_nervous.html>.

7. Kromer W. Endogenous and exogenous opioids in the control of gastrointestinal motility and secretion. *Pharmacol Rev* 1988;40:121-162.

8. Reisine T, Paternak G. Opioid analgesic and antagonists. In Hardman JG, Limbird LE, Gilman AG (eds.), *Goodman & Gilman's The pharmacological basis of therapeutics*. New York: McGraw-Hill, 1996:521-555.

9. Kromer W. The current status of opioid research on gastrointestinal motility. *Life Sci* 1989;44:579-589.

10. Manara L, Bianchetti A. The central and peripheral influences of opioids on gastrointestinal propulsion. *Annu Rev Pharmacol Toxicol* 1985;25:249-273.

11. Nishiwaki H, Saitoh N, Nishio H, Takeuchi T, Hata F. Relationship between inhibitory effect of endogenous opioid via mu-receptors and muscarinic auto-inhibition in acetylcholine release from myenteric plexus of guinea pig ileum. *Jpn J Pharmacol* 1998;77:279-286.

12. Nishimura E, Buchan AM, McIntosh CH. Autoradiographic localization of mu- and delta-type opioid receptors in the gastrointestinal tract of the rat and guinea pig. *Gastroenterology* 1986;91:1084-1094.

13. De Luca A, Coupar IM. Insights into opioid action in the intestinal tract. *Pharmacol Ther* 1996;69:103-115.

14. Bueno L, Fioramonti J, Honde C, Fargeas MJ, Primi MP. Central and peripheral control of gastrointestinal and colonic motility by endogenous opiates in conscious dogs. *Gastroenterology* 1985;88:549-556.

15. Parolaro D, Sala M, Gori E. Effect of intracerebroventricular administration of morphine upon intestinal motility in rat and its antagonism with naloxone. *Eur J Pharmacol* 1977;46:329-338.

16. Porreca F, Cowan A, Raffa RB, Tallarida RJ. Ketazocines and morphine: Effects on gastrointestinal transit after central and peripheral administration. *Life Sci* 1983;32:1785-1790.

17. Porreca F, Mosberg HI, Hurst R, Hruby VJ, Burks TF. Roles of mu, delta and kappa opioid receptors in spinal and supraspinal mediation of gastrointestinal transit effects and hot-plate analgesia in the mouse. *J Pharmacol Exp Ther* 1984; 230:341-348.

18. Parolaro D, Crema G, Sala M, Santagostino A, Giagnoni G, Gori E. Intestinal effect and analgesia: Evidence for different involvement of opioid receptor subtypes in periaqueductal gray matter. *Eur J Pharmacol* 1986;120:95-99.

19. Ward SJ, Takemori AE. Relative involvement of receptor subtypes in opioid-induced inhibition of intestinal motility in mice. *Life Sci* 1982;31:1267-1270.

20. Manara L, Bianchi G, Ferretti P, Tavani A. Inhibition of gastrointestinal transit by morphine in rats results primarily from direct drug action on gut opioid sites. *J Pharmacol Exp Ther* 1986;237:945-949.

21. Shook JE, Lemcke PK, Gehrig CA, Hruby VJ, Burks TF. Antidiarrheal properties of supraspinal mu and delta and peripheral mu, delta and kappa opioid receptors: Inhibition of diarrhea without constipation. *J Pharmacol Exp Ther* 1989; 249:83-90.

22. Shook JE, Pelton JT, Hruby VJ, Burks TF. Peptide opioid antagonist separates peripheral and central opioid antitransit effects. *J Pharmacol Exp Ther* 1987; 243:492-500.

23. Thompson AR, Ray JB. The importance of opioid tolerance: A therapeutic paradox. *J Am Coll Surg* 2003;196:321-324.

24. Cherubini E, North RA. Mu and kappa opioids inhibit transmitter release by different mechanisms. *Proc Natl Acad Sci USA* 1985;82:1860-1863.

25. Nishiwaki H, Saitoh N, Nishio H, Takeuch T, Hata F. Possible role of potassium channels in mu-receptor-mediated inhibition and muscarinic autoinhibition in acetylcholine release from myenteric plexus of guinea pig ileum. *Jpn J Pharmacol* 2000;82:343-349.

26. Hare B, Lipman A. Uses and misuses of medications in the treatment of chronic pain. In Hare B, Fine P (eds.), *Chronic pain, problems in anesthesia.* Philadelphia: JB Lippincott Co.; 1990:577-594.

27. Uhl GR, Sora I, Wang Z. The mu opiate receptor as a candidate gene for pain: Polymorphisms, variations in expression, nociception, and opiate responses. *Proc Natl Acad Sci USA* 1999;96:7752-7755.

28. Inturrisi CE. Clinical pharmacology of opioids for pain. *Clin J Pain* 2002; 18:S3-S13.

29. Peracchia F, Bianchi G, Fiocchi R, Petrillo P, Tavani A, Manara L. Central and peripheral inhibition of gastrointestinal transit in rats: Narcotics differ substantially by acting at either or both levels. *J Pharm Pharmacol* 1984;36:699-701.

30. Nugent M, Davis C, Brooks D, Ahmedzai SH. Long-term observations of patients receiving transdermal fentanyl after a randomized trial. *J Pain Symptom Manage* 2001;21:385-391.

31. Choi YS, Billings JA. Opioid antagonists: A review of their role in palliative care, focusing on use in opioid-related constipation. *J Pain Symptom Manage* 2002;24:71-90.

32. Yuan C. Methylnaltrexone: Investigation of clinical applications. *Drug Development Research* 2000;50:133-141.

33. Schmidt WK. Alvimopan (ADL 8-2698) is a novel peripheral opioid antagonist. *Am J Surg* 2001;182:27S-38S.

Chapter 2

Pathophysiology of Opioid-Induced Bowel Dysfunction

Sangeeta R. Mehendale
Chun-Su Yuan

Opioids have been used extensively as potent analgesics for the treatment of moderate to severe pain caused by cancer or surgery.[1-3] Although opioids offer excellent pain relief, their use is associated with adverse bowel-related effects such as constipation, nausea, and vomiting, which severely compromise patients' quality of life.[4] Reducing the severity of these adverse effects is of utmost importance for patients to experience the benefits of opioid analgesics. Since opioids mediate their gastrointestinal and analgesic effects through the same classes of receptors, namely, mu, delta, and kappa (discussed earlier in Chapter 1), it has been challenging to dissociate their beneficial analgesic effects from the untoward gastrointestinal effects. This chapter reviews the underlying pathophysiological mechanisms of specific gastrointestinal adverse effects of opioids. The role of endogenous opioids in certain gastrointestinal diseases is also discussed.

GASTROINTESTINAL DYSFUNCTION CAUSED BY EXOGENOUS OPIOIDS

Nausea and Vomiting

Nausea and vomiting are important adverse effects of opioid administration. Nausea is an essential component of the vomiting sensation, yet it may occur exclusively. Of the patients being treated with opioids, 8 to 35 percent patients reported nausea while 14 to 40 percent patients suffered from vomiting.[5,6]

Opioids act centrally at the chemoreceptor trigger zone (area postrema), triggering emetic mechanisms mediated by the vomiting center. The area postrema is essential for opioid-induced vomiting, as demonstrated by animal studies in which ablation of the area postrema eliminates the emetic response to opioids.[7,8] The blood-brain barrier in the area postrema is not complete and therefore, pharmacologically, is considered a peripheral compartment. The emetic effect of morphine can therefore be blocked by methylnaltrexone, a quaternary mu opioid antagonist with peripherally restricted action.[9] Delta receptors could also partly mediate the emetic response since enkephalin receptors have been demonstrated in the chemoreceptor trigger zone in dogs.[10] Interestingly, at higher doses specific opioids also act as antiemetics by acting downstream from the area postrema on the vomiting center.[8,11]

In addition to the effect of opioid agonists on the chemoreceptor trigger zone, the other central actions of opioids result in inhibition of gastric motility and delay in gastric emptying, with a predominant mu receptor involvement.[12,13] Morphine, even at lower doses, slows gastric emptying in humans.[14] Mu receptor agonists also relax the lower esophageal sphincter (LES) and increase the probability of reflux in monkeys and humans.[15] Some studies report LES contraction instead of relaxation and could represent a direct myogenic action of opioids on the sphincter smooth muscle cells.[16] Like morphine, delta agonists also cause delayed gastric emptying.[17,18] These gastric effects of opioid agonists could contribute to nausea and vomiting by activating gastrointestinal mechanoreceptors that convey signals to the brainstem vomiting center via vagae afferents.[19] The vagal input to the vomiting center may only be complementary since in ferrets, loperamide-induced emesis (subcutaneous administration) was not altered by abdominal vagotomy.[8]

Several therapeutic and experimental alternatives have been proposed to reduce the incidence of opioid-induced nausea and vomiting. Used intrathecally, highly lipophilic agents such as lofentanil are rapidly absorbed locally and may delay the centrally mediated adverse effects of opioids.[20] Substituting opioids that induce emesis with kappa agonists has been proposed for analgesia, since kappa agonists show evidence of antiemetic activity only without any emetic activity.[7] Combining opioids with other drugs to improve analgesia and reduce nausea and vomiting is also a consideration. In one clinical study simultaneous treatment with fluoxetine, a selective serotonin reuptake inhibitor, marginally improved morphine-induced analgesia and reduced morphine-induced nausea, suggesting that serotonin and morphine interact in pain and gastrointestinal regulation.[21] However, since serotonin itself can induce nausea and vomiting,[22,23] additional studies are required to optimize the interaction between the two drugs to avoid nausea.

Constipation

Constipation, a major symptom of bowel malfunction, manifests as straining, difficulty in evacuation of stools, hardened dried stools, and abdominal distension.[24] Opioid-induced constipation is found in 40 to 50 percent of patients who are treated with morphine,[24,25] making it a significant adverse effect of opioids.

Opioid-induced constipation is seen even with a single administration of morphine.[26,27] The dose of opioids that induces constipation is much smaller than that required for analgesia; thus, using lower doses of opioids will not prevent constipation.[28,29] With repeated exposure to morphine, tolerance to constipation does not develop as it does for other effects, such as analgesia.[30,31] Tolerance development may be linked to the existence of subtypes of mu receptors that mediate various pharmacological actions.[30,32] It appears that tolerance develops more readily to mu-1-dependent actions than to non-mu-1-dependent actions. Another hypothesis suggests that P-glycoprotein (the drug efflux protein) up-regulation is required for tolerance development. Morphine induces P-glycoprotein up-regulation in the brain, but it does not up-regulate intestinal P-glycoprotein.[33]

Although centrally administered opioid peptides influence colonic activity, the opioid-induced peripheral regulation of colonic function appears to be more important. Prolonged retention of morphine in the intestinal tissue following intravenous administration suggests that it may exert local effects on the enteric nervous system and intestines.[24,34] The overall constipating effect of opioids results from reduced intestinal motility and increased fluid reabsorption in the intestines. The increased contractile activity of the circular muscle layer of colon results in frequent segmenting, nonpropulsive contractions, and increased intestinal transit time.[24]

Mu agonists decrease intestinal motility when administered centrally, spinally, or peripherally.[35,36] Central delta and kappa receptors mediate inhibition of colonic motility in different species.[36,37] When administered intrathecally, kappa opioid receptor agonists also are effective in inhibiting intestinal motility.[38] In cats, prejunctional inhibitory delta receptors, present on the sacral parasympathetic outflow to the colon, caused inhibition of colonic activity.[39] Thus, when opioids are administered centrally or intrathecally they mediate inhibition of colonic motility irrespective of the class of opioid receptor evaluated.

The effects of peripherally administered opioids on the large intestine vary according to the species and the segment of the colon studied.[37,40,41] In rabbits, peripherally administered delta and kappa agonists decreased colonic activity;[40] however, kappa agonists did not inhibit intestinal transit in rats,[42] suggesting a species-dependent distribution of specific opioid receptors. Similarly, in guinea pigs, an orally administered kappa agonist delayed the intestinal transit; in rats no effect occurred.[41,43] Within the intestine, specific opioid receptors are found on the circular muscles but not on the longitudinal muscles. Such a receptor distribution results in nonpropulsive contractions caused by circular muscles, typical of opioid-induced bowel dysfunction. The inhibitory effect of opioid agonists on the ileocecal sphincter, defecation reflexes, and secretions also contribute to opioid-induced constipation.[24,44]

Understanding the pathophysiological mechanisms of opioid-induced constipation has led to several experimental therapeutic possibilities for reducing the slow gastrointestinal transit. The various possibilities are enumerated.

Newer Opioid Compounds

With newer compounds such as dihydroetorphine hydrochloride the incidence of constipation is reduced significantly.[45] Opioids with partial antagonistic actions, selective peripheral opioid antagonists, and highly lipid-soluble opioid agonists used in spinal anesthesia have been proposed to minimize the central effects of opioids during spinal anesthesia.[20] The last two chapters of this book discuss the current status of two selective peripheral opioid antagonists, methylnal-trexone and alvimopan, which are under clinical investigation.

Route of Administration

When the transdermal fentanyl patch was compared with oral morphine, fentanyl produced reduced constipation as gauged by the reduction in laxatives consumed by patients in each group. Thus change in route of administration of this lipophilic opioid agonist may minimize constipation by reducing the peripheral effects while maintaining analgesic efficacy.[46-48]

Combination with Other Medications

Opioids used in combination with other classes of drugs, such as alpha-2 adrenoceptor agonists that complement their antinociceptive activity, could help maintain adequate analgesia at lower opioid doses.[20] Use of adjuncts such as selective serotonin reuptake inhibitors can increase morphine-induced analgesia while countering constipation by increasing concentration of serotonin in the gut (increased serotonin could however stimulate nausea and vomiting).[49] The use of adjuvant drugs with morphine such as nonsteroidal anti-inflammatory drugs, antipsychotics, and benzodiazepines, which reduce pain through nonopioid pathways, has been suggested to reduce constipation.[50] Nitric oxide precursor, which reverses morphine-induced constipation by acting locally in the gut, has been proposed to combat opioid-induced constipation without interference with its central analgesic activity.[51]

Postoperative Ileus

Postoperative ileus is characterized as a functional inhibition of the propulsive activity of the intestines following surgery.[52] Although postoperative ileus is more commonly associated with abdominal surgery, it occurs with other surgeries as well.[53,54] An "uncomplicated ileus" is caused by the neurohumoral stimulation that occurs during surgery and resolves spontaneously two to three days later.[55] A more severe form, paralytic postoperative ileus, lasts for more than three days after surgery.[55]

The pathophysiological factors that cause postoperative ileus can be endogenous (neurohumoral response) or exogenous (anesthesia, opioids).[55,56] The contribution of endogenous factors depends on the level of pain and the degree of abdominal manipulation.[57,58] Increased sympathetic activation resulting from the stressful stimulus of surgery is a significant cause of reduced gut motility, which is aggravated by other gut-related humoral factors, including endogenous opioids, vasoactive intestinal peptide (VIP), substance P, calcitonin gene-related peptide (CGRP), and nitric oxide.[55,56] Levels of inflammatory mediators and cytokines are also elevated in the gut and have been implicated in the reduced gastrointestinal motility following abdominal surgery.[55,56] Exogenous factors such as general anesthetics and opioid analgesics can worsen postoperative ileus. These factors may act simultaneously or during different phases. The exact contribution of each factor is not clear, thus making management of the condition challenging.

When opioids are used postoperatively for analgesia, administration of mu receptor antagonists with selective peripheral action can reduce the severity of postoperative ileus. Mu receptor antagonists, such as methylnaltrexone, can inhibit opioid gut effect without compromising the central analgesic effects of morphine or initiating opioid withdrawal.[59,60] Another mu opioid receptor antagonist ADL 8-2698 (alvimopan) shortened the median time to passage of first flatus, the median time to the first bowel movement, and the length of hospital stay for patients who had abdominal surgery and were treated with opioids for postoperative analgesia.[61] It is important to note that although mu receptor antagonists partly reverse the bowel dysfunction caused by opioids and may reverse the actions of endogenous opioids, they do not totally eliminate postsurgical bowel dysfunction. The treatment of postoperative ileus, therefore, needs to be multimodal.[55]

Kappa receptor agonists, rather than opioid antagonists, are being tested as treatment for postoperative ileus.[62-64] One cause of postoperative ileus is proposed to be the activation of an inhibitory nervous reflex pathway.[63] Kappa agonists, which were shown to increase the threshold of activation of the afferent limb of the inhibitory reflex,[65] could thereby prevent reduction of bowel movements.

ROLE OF ENDOGENOUS OPIOIDS
IN NORMAL AND IMPAIRED GUT FUNCTION

Endogenous Opioid System of the Gut

As discussed in Chapter 1, the major opioid peptide classes—endorphins, enkephalins, and dynorphins—are natural agonists for opioid receptors mu, delta, and kappa, respectively.[66] Few other endogenously found opioid peptides such as endomorphins and nociceptin also exert gastrointestinal effects.[66-68] In the gastrointestinal wall, the opioid receptors are present in the submucosal plexus and the myenteric plexus, on the intestinal smooth muscle cells (circular layer), and on the enterocytes.[27,69]

Endogenous opioid peptides are found in miniscule quantities in the neurons of the enteric nervous system ranging from 10^{-10} to 10^{-12} mol·g^{-1} of intestinal tissue.[27] These peptides affect motility, secretions, and the reflex activity of the gut. They interact extensively with several other locally released neurohumoral mediators, including acetylcholine, vasoactive intestinal peptide (VIP), somatostatin, serotonin, calcitonin gene-related peptide (CGRP), and substance P, to exert control over the reflex activity in the gut.[27,70,71] The isolated effects of these mediators are enumerated in Table 1.1 of Chapter 1.

Our understanding of the role of endogenous opioids in the gut has been derived mainly from examining the effects of opioid antagonists on gut function.[26,27] Several studies have also evaluated gut responses to exogenously administered opioid agonists. But the observations from these studies reflect the pharmacological effects of endogenous opioids rather than their physiological functions. The use of knockout mice models for opioid receptors in evaluating the physiological role of endogenous opioid peptides in gastrointestinal function is only beginning.[72,73]

Endogenous Opioids in Peristalsis

In vitro experiments using intestinal segments from various species demonstrated that opioid antagonists increase the frequency and amplitude of distension-mediated peristaltic contractions and decrease the duration of peristalsis-free periods.[27] In addition, release of endogenous opioids is reduced during peristalsis, suggesting that opioids inhibit peristalsis.[74-76] Conversely, it could also suggest that opioid release is attenuated during peristalsis. Opioids inhibit release of the excitatory neurotransmitter acetylcholine in the enteric nervous system. This could represent one of the mechanisms by which endogenous opioids reduce gut motility.[76-78] The effects of opioids are further complicated by the fact that the neurogenic action of endogenous opioids seems to inhibit the overall gastrointestinal motility, while direct effects of opioids on the circular muscle layer result in contractions. Stimulation of opioid receptors located on the circular muscle layer[24,69] result in segmental contractions of the circular muscle layer. Thus, the endogenous opioids appear to reduce the overall gut motility with periodic segmental contractions and may represent the gut activity between meals or during fasting (described in Chapter 1). When opioids are administered pharmacologically, however, an exaggerated neurogenic and myogenic effect results in increased nonpropulsive segmental contractions, leading to slower intestinal transit and constipation.

When peristalsis is initiated by a radial stretch or a bolus of food, endogenous opioids function in an orchestrated manner with other neurotransmitters to propel the bolus aborally.[79] Release of endogenous opioid peptides is decreased during the descending relaxation of intestinal muscles (described in Chapter 1) distal to the bolus. This in turn results in reduced constraining influence on VIP release in the circular muscles, which mediates circular muscle relaxation.[70,78] Release of nitric oxide with VIP also relaxes the circular muscles during the descending relaxation phase.[70] The opposite sequence of events, caused by release of opioid peptides, occurs during the complementary ascending contraction phase of peristalsis. The circular muscles contract in a constricting fashion proximal to the bolus to propel it in the aboral direction. The circular muscle contraction during this phase is the net effect of the direct myogenic and indirect neurogenic action (inhibition of VIP release) of opioids. Opioid release may be regulated partly by somatostatin.[70,77] The somatostatin release may in turn be stimulated by serotonin and CGRP released in response to a food bolus.[71] Clearly, the control of reflex gastrointestinal motility is a complex but a well-coordinated phenomenon involving multiple mediators.

Endogenous Opioids in Fluid and Electrolyte Absorption

Endogenous opioids also exert their effects on fluid absorption and ion secretion in the intestine. Some evidence suggests that endogenous opioids exert a tonic inhibition of net fluid secretion.[80] Administration of naloxone in a guinea pig intestinal model increased chloride secretion, suggesting the inhibitory influence of endogenous opioids.[81] The significance of the antisecretory effects under physiological conditions is not yet clear.

Imbalance of Endogenous Opioids in Gastrointestinal Diseases

Imbalance of endogenous opioid peptides has been proposed to contribute in the pathogenesis of some diseases such as idiopathic constipation, irritable bowel syndrome, achalasia, Hirschsprung's disease, and Crohn's disease.[27] However, as described earlier, the control of gastrointestinal function by endogenous opioid peptides is quite complex. Thus, causality of a disease exclusively owing to deficiency of endogenous peptides is not possible to ascertain. Also, it is not possible to evaluate whether the altered opioid mechanisms in some gastrointestinal pathologies are the cause or the effect of the pathology, because other endogenous mediators may affect the activity of endogenous opioids.[70,82-84]

Idiopathic Constipation

Alterations in the endogenous opioid peptides in the gastrointestinal tract have been used to explain the pathophysiology of slow gut transit in idiopathic constipation. The role of opioids in idiopathic constipation is supported by the fact that naloxone speeds up colonic transit in healthy volunteers,[26] but in patients with idiopathic constipation results were ambiguous: one study found that constipation was reversed with naloxone and another study found no benefit with naloxone or nalmefene.[85,86]

There is also ambiguity in the reports of enkephalin content in the colonic tissue from patients with slow transit constipation. In two studies, enkephalin activity was found to be reduced in the circular muscle of the large intestine of patients with slow transit constipation.[87,88] In another study, no differences were found in the enkephalin and dynorphin levels in the colon specimens from slow transit constipation.[89] Similarly, the met-enkephalin content of colon specimens from patients with chronic constipation was not different from normal.[90] However, both these studies demonstrated alterations in other mediators, such as CGRP and VIP. These observations suggest that multiple neurohumoral mediators, including endogenous opioids, may be involved in the pathophysiology of idiopathic constipation.

Irritable Bowel Syndrome

Irritable bowel syndrome (IBS) is characterized by abdominal pain, bloating, and disturbed defecation (constipation or diarrhea) in the absence of other medical conditions with similar presentations. In patients with IBS release of endogenous opioids may be diminished in response to aversive visceral stimulation.[91]

Opioid agonists are used in the management of IBS.[92] Kappa receptor agonists such as fedotozine are used as visceral analgesics and mu agonists that are not systemically absorbed, such as loperamide, are given for treating diarrhea.[92] In a clinical trial for treatment of IBS with constipation, naloxone was effective in reducing constipation and thus improving the quality of life.[93]

In summary, a better understanding of the pathophysiological mechanisms of opioid-induced bowel dysfunction has led to the development of newer opioid analgesics and improved regimens, resulting in reduced gastrointestinal adverse effects. The involvement of endogenous opioids in certain gastrointestinal disorders of motility and secretion is less clear and may represent only a part of the overall pathophysiological process.

NOTES

1. O'Mahony S, Coyle N, Payne R. Current management of opioid-related side effects. *Oncology (Huntingt)* 2001;15:61-73, 77; discussion 77-78, 80-82.

2. Portenoy RK. Management of common opioid side effects during long-term therapy of cancer pain. *Ann Acad Med Singapore* 1994;23:160-170.

3. Holder KA, Dougherty TB, Porche VH, Chiang JS. Postoperative pain management. *Int Anesthesiol Clin* 1998;36:71-86.

4. Thorpe DM. Management of opioid-induced constipation. *Curr Pain Headache Rep* 2001;5:237-240.

5. Campora E, Merlini L, Pace M, Bruzzone M, Luzzani M, Gottlieb A, Rosso R. The incidence of narcotic-induced emesis. *J Pain Symptom Manage* 1991;6:428-430.

6. Aparasu R, McCoy RA, Weber C, Mair D, Parasuraman TV. Opioid-induced emesis among hospitalized nonsurgical patients: Effect on pain and quality of life. *J Pain Symptom Manage* 1999;18:280-288.

7. Blancquaert JP, Lefebvre RA, Willems JL. Emetic and antiemetic effects of opioids in the dog. *Eur J Pharmacol* 1986;128:143-150.

8. Bhandari P, Bingham S, Andrews PL. The neuropharmacology of loperamide-induced emesis in the ferret: The role of the area postrema, vagus, opiate and 5-HT3 receptors. *Neuropharmacology* 1992;31:735-742.

9. Foss JF, Bass AS, Goldberg LI. Dose-related antagonism of the emetic effect of morphine by methylnaltrexone in dogs. *J Clin Pharmacol* 1993;33:747-751.

10. Bhargava KP, Dixit KS, Gupta YK. Enkephalin receptors in the emetic chemoreceptor trigger zone of the dog. *Br J Pharmacol* 1981;72:471-475.

11. Foss JF, Yuan CS, Roizen MF, Goldberg LI. Prevention of apomorphine- or cisplatin-induced emesis in the dog by a combination of methylnaltrexone and morphine. *Cancer Chemother Pharmacol* 1998;42:287-291.

12. Bueno L, Fioramonti J. Action of opiates on gastrointestinal function. *Baillieres Clin Gastroenterol* 1988;2:123-139.

13. Improta G, Broccardo M. Effect of selective mu 1, mu 2 and delta 2 opioid receptor agonists on gastric functions in the rat. *Neuropharmacology* 1994;33:977-981.

14. Yuan CS, Foss JF, O'Connor M, Roizen MF, Moss J. Effects of low-dose morphine on gastric emptying in healthy volunteers. *J Clin Pharmacol* 1998;38:1017-1020.

15. Hall AW, Moossa AR, Clark J, Cooley GR, Skinner DB. The effects of premedication drugs on the lower oesophageal high pressure zone and reflux status of rhesus monkeys and man. *Gut* 1975;16:347-352.

16. Strombeck DR, Harrold D. Effect of gastrin, histamine, serotonin, and adrenergic amines on gastroesophageal sphincter pressure in the dog. *Am J Vet Res* 1985;46:1684-1690.

17. Sullivan SN, Lamki L, Corcoran P. Inhibition of gastric emptying by enkephalin analogue. *Lancet* 1981;2:86-87.

18. Sullivan SN. The pharmacologic effects of naloxone and an enkephalin analogue on human upper gastrointestinal motility and secretion. In Fraioli F, Isidori A, Mazzetti M (eds.), *Opioid peptides in the periphery.* New York: Elsevier Science Publishers; 1984:213-224.

19. Andrews PL, Wood KL. Vagally mediated gastric motor and emetic reflexes evoked by stimulation of the antral mucosa in anaesthetized ferrets. *J Physiol* 1988;395:1-16.

20. Foldes FF. Pain control with intrathecally and peridurally administered opioids and other drugs. *Anaesthesiol Reanim* 1991;16:287-298.

21. Erjavec MK, Coda BA, Nguyen Q, Donaldson G, Risler L, Shen DD. Morphine-fluoxetine interactions in healthy volunteers: Analgesia and side effects. *J Clin Pharmacol* 2000;40:1286-1295.

22. DeVane CL. Immediate-release versus controlled-release formulations: Pharmacokinetics of newer antidepressants in relation to nausea. *J Clin Psychiatry* 2003;64 Suppl 18:14-19.

23. Hasler WL. Serotonin receptor physiology: Relation to emesis. *Dig Dis Sci* 1999;44:108S-113S.

24. Choi YS, Billings JA. Opioid antagonists: A review of their role in palliative care, focusing on use in opioid-related constipation. *J Pain Symptom Manage* 2002;24:71-90.

25. Pappagallo M. Incidence, prevalence, and management of opioid bowel dysfunction. *Am J Surg* 2001;182:11S-18S.

26. Kaufman PN, Krevsky B, Malmud LS, Maurer AH, Somers MB, Siegel JA, Fisher RS. Role of opiate receptors in the regulation of colonic transit. *Gastroenterology* 1988;94:1351-1356.

27. Kromer W. Endogenous and exogenous opioids in the control of gastrointestinal motility and secretion. *Pharmacol Rev* 1988;40:121-162.

28. Shook JE, Pelton JT, Hruby VJ, Burks TF. Peptide opioid antagonist separates peripheral and central opioid antitransit effects. *J Pharmacol Exp Ther* 1987; 243:492-500.

29. Shook JE, Lemcke PK, Gehrig CA, Hruby VJ, Burks TF. Antidiarrheal properties of supraspinal mu and delta and peripheral mu, delta and kappa opioid receptors: Inhibition of diarrhea without constipation. *J Pharmacol Exp Ther* 1989; 249:83-90.

30. Ling GS, Paul D, Simantov R, Pasternak GW. Differential development of acute tolerance to analgesia, respiratory depression, gastrointestinal transit and hormone release in a morphine infusion model. *Life Sci* 1989;45:1627-1636.

31. Thompson AR, Ray JB. The importance of opioid tolerance: A therapeutic paradox. *J Am Coll Surg* 2003;196:321-324.

32. Pasternak GW. Incomplete cross tolerance and multiple mu opioid peptide receptors. *Trends Pharmacol Sci* 2001;22:67-70.

33. Tan-No K, Niijima F, Nakagawasai O, Sato T, Satoh S, Tadano T. Development of tolerance to the inhibitory effect of loperamide on gastrointestinal transit in mice. *Eur J Pharm Sci* 2003;20:357-363.

34. Yuan CS, Foss JF, O'Connor M, Toledano A, Roizen MF, Moss J. Methylnaltrexone prevents morphine-induced delay in oral-cecal transit time without affecting analgesia: A double-blind randomized placebo-controlled trial. *Clin Pharmacol Ther* 1996;59:469-475.

35. Sugahara S, Rosen M, Juniper CJ, Johnston KR, Davies RL. Effects of intrathecal and intraperitoneal morphine on gastrointestinal motility in the rat. *Eur J Anaesthesiol* 1992;9:341-346.

36. Raffa RB, Mathiasen JR, Jacoby HI. Colonic bead expulsion time in normal and mu-opioid receptor deficient (CXBK) mice following central (ICV) administration of mu- and delta-opioid agonists. *Life Sci* 1987;41:2229-2234.

37. Bardon T, Ruckebusch Y. Comparative effects of opiate agonists on proximal and distal colonic motility in dogs. *Eur J Pharmacol* 1985;110:329-334.

38. Shukla VK, Turndorf H, Bansinath M. Pertussis and cholera toxins modulate kappa-opioid receptor agonists-induced hypothermia and gut inhibition. *Eur J Pharmacol* 1995;292:293-299.

39. Kennedy C, Krier J. Delta-opioid receptors mediate inhibition of fast excitatory postsynaptic potentials in cat parasympathetic colonic ganglia. *Br J Pharmacol* 1987;92:437-443.

40. Pairet M, Ruckebusch Y. Opioid receptor agonists in the rabbit colon: Comparison of in vivo and in vitro studies. *Life Sci* 1984;35:1653-1658.

41. Culpepper-Morgan J, Kreek MJ, Holt PR, LaRoche D, Zhang J, O'Bryan L. Orally administered kappa as well as mu opiate agonists delay gastrointestinal transit time in the guinea pig. *Life Sci* 1988;42:2073-2077.

42. Tavani A, Gambino MC, Petrillo P. The opioid kappa-selective compound U-50,488H does not inhibit intestinal propulsion in rats. *J Pharm Pharmacol* 1984; 36:343-344.

43. Culpepper-Morgan JA, Holt PR, LaRoche D, Kreek MJ. Orally administered opioid antagonists reverse both mu and kappa opioid agonist delay of gastrointestinal transit in the guinea pig. *Life Sci* 1995;56:1187-1192.

44. Ouyang A, Vos P, Cohen S. Sites of action of mu-, kappa- and sigma-opiate receptor agonists at the feline ileocecal sphincter. *Am J Physiol* 1988;254:G224-G231.

45. Ohmori S, Morimoto Y. Dihydroetorphine: A potent analgesic: Pharmacology, toxicology, pharmacokinetics, and clinical effects. *CNS Drug Rev* 2002;8:391-404.

46. Grond S, Radbruch L, Lehmann KA. Clinical pharmacokinetics of transdermal opioids: Focus on transdermal fentanyl. *Clin Pharmacokinet* 2000; 38:59-89.

47. Radbruch L, Sabatowski R, Loick G, Kulbe C, Kasper M, Grond S, Lehmann KA. Constipation and the use of laxatives: A comparison between transdermal fentanyl and oral morphine. *Palliat Med* 2000;14:111-119.

48. Jeal W, Benfield P. Transdermal fentanyl: A review of its pharmacological properties and therapeutic efficacy in pain control. *Drugs* 1997;53:109-138.

49. Ise Y, Katayama S, Hirano M, Aoki T, Narita M, Suzuki T. Effects of fluvoxamine on morphine-induced inhibition of gastrointestinal transit, antinociception and hyperlocomotion in mice. *Neurosci Lett* 2001;299:29-32.

50. Goldstein FJ. Adjuncts to opioid therapy. *J Am Osteopath Assoc.* 2002; 102:S15-S21.

51. Calignano A, Moncada S, Di Rosa M. Endogenous nitric oxide modulates morphine-induced constipation. *Biochem Biophys Res Commun* 1991;181:889-893.

52. Livingston EH, Passaro EP, Jr. Postoperative ileus. *Dig Dis Sci* 1990;35:121-132.

53. Welling RE, Rath R, Albers JE, Glaser RS. Gastrointestinal complications after cardiac surgery. *Arch Surg* 1986;121:1178-1180.

54. Benacker SA. Managing quality on an orthopedic service: Ileus in the lumbar spinal fusion patient. *J Healthc Qual* 1993;15:17-20.

55. Luckey A, Livingston E, Tache Y. Mechanisms and treatment of postoperative ileus. *Arch Surg* 2003;138:206-214.

56. Kurz A, Sessler DI. Opioid-induced bowel dysfunction: Pathophysiology and potential new therapies. *Drugs* 2003;63:649-671.

57. Le Blanc-Louvry I, Coquerel A, Koning E, Maillot C, Ducrotte P. Operative stress response is reduced after laparoscopic compared to open cholecystectomy: The relationship with postoperative pain and ileus. *Dig Dis Sci* 2000;45:1703-1713.

58. De Winter BY, Boeckxstaens GE, De Man JG, Moreels TG, Herman AG, Pelckmans PA. Effect of adrenergic and nitrergic blockade on experimental ileus in rats. *Br J Pharmacol* 1997;120:464-468.

59. Yuan CS, Foss JF. Antagonism of gastrointestinal opioid effects. *Reg Anesth Pain Med* 2000;25:639-642.

60. Foss JF. A review of the potential role of methylnaltrexone in opioid bowel dysfunction. *Am J Surg* 2001;182:19S-26S.

61. Taguchi A, Sharma N, Saleem RM, Sessler DI, Carpenter RL, Seyedsadr M, Kurz A. Selective postoperative inhibition of gastrointestinal opioid receptors. *N Engl J Med* 2001;345:935-940.

62. Delvaux M. Pharmacology and clinical experience with fedotozine. *Expert Opin Investig Drugs* 2001;10:97-110.

63. De Winter BY, Boeckxstaens GE, De Man JG, Moreels TG, Herman AG, Pelckmans PA. Effects of mu- and kappa-opioid receptors on postoperative ileus in rats. *Eur J Pharmacol* 1997;339:63-67.

64. Riviere PJ, Pascaud X, Chevalier E, Junien JL. Fedotozine reversal of peritoneal-irritation-induced ileus in rats. Possible peripheral action on sensory afferents. *J Pharmacol Exp Ther* 1994;270:846-850.

65. Sengupta JN, Su X, Gebhart GF. Kappa, but not mu or delta, opioids attenuate responses to distention of afferent fibers innervating the rat colon. *Gastroenterology* 1996;111:968-980.

66. Kromer W. Endogenous opioids, the enteric nervous system and gut motility. *Dig Dis* 1990;8:361-373.

67. Okada Y, Tsuda Y, Bryant SD, Lazarus LH. Endomorphins and related opioid peptides. *Vitam Horm* 2002;65:257-279.

68. Osinski MA, Pampusch MS, Murtaugh MP, Brown DR. Cloning, expression and functional role of a nociceptin/orphanin FQ receptor in the porcine gastrointestinal tract. *Eur J Pharmacol* 1999;365:281-289.

69. Bitar KN, Makhlouf GM. Selective presence of opiate receptors on intestinal circular muscle cells. *Life Sci* 1985;37:1545-1550.

70. Grider JR. Interplay of somatostatin, opioid, and GABA neurons in the regulation of the peristaltic reflex. *Am J Physiol* 1994;267:G696-G701.

71. Grider JR. Neurotransmitters mediating the intestinal peristaltic reflex in the mouse. *J Pharmacol Exp Ther* 2003;307:460-467.

72. Roy S, Liu HC, Loh HH. mu-opioid receptor-knockout mice: The role of mu-opioid receptor in gastrointestinal transit. *Brain Res Mol Brain Res* 1998;56:281-283.

73. Mitolo-Chieppa D, Natale L, Marasciulo FL, De Salvatore G, Mitolo CI, Siro-Brigiani G, Renna G, De Salvia MA. Involvement of kappa-opioid receptors in peripheral response to nerve stimulation in kappa-opioid receptor knockout mice. *Auton Autacoid Pharmacol* 2002;22:233-239.

74. Clark SJ, Smith TW. Peristalsis abolishes the release of methionine-enkephalin from guinea-pig ileum in vitro. *Eur J Pharmacol* 1981;70:421-424.

75. Clark SJ, Smith TW. The release of Met-enkephalin from the guinea-pig ileum at rest and during peristaltic activity. *Life Sci* 1983;33 Suppl 1:465-468.

76. Kromer W, Hollt V, Schmidt H, Herz A. Release of immunoreactive-dynorphin from the isolated guinea-pig small intestine is reduced during peristaltic activity. *Neurosci Lett* 1981;25:53-56.

77. Andrews PL, Widdicombe J. *Pathophysiology of the gut and airways: An introduction.* Chapel Hill, NC: Portland Press; 1993.

78. Grider JR, Makhlouf GM. Role of opioid neurons in the regulation of intestinal peristalsis. *Am J Physiol* 1987;253:G226-G231.

79. Kromer W. Gastrointestinal effects of opioids. In Herz A (ed.), *Handbook of experimental pharmacology. Opioids II.* Berlin: Springer-Verlag; 1993.

80. Fogel R, Kaplan RB. Role of enkephalins in regulation of basal intestinal water and ion absorption in the rat. *Am J Physiol* 1984;246:G386-G392.

81. Kachur JF, Miller RJ. Characterization of the opiate receptor in the guinea-pig ileal mucosa. *Eur J Pharmacol* 1982;81:177-183.

82. Garzon J, Hollt V, Schulz R, Herz A. Excitatory neuropeptides activate opioid mechanisms in the guinea pig ileum. *Neuropeptides* 1985;5:583-586.

83. Garzon J, Hollt V, Herz A. Cholecystokinin octapeptide activates an opioid mechanism in the guinea-pig ileum: A possible role for substance P. *Eur J Pharmacol* 1987;136:361-370.

84. Grider JR. Reciprocal activity of longitudinal and circular muscle during intestinal peristaltic reflex. *Am J Physiol Gastrointest Liver Physiol* 2003;284:G768-G775.

85. Kreek MJ, Schaefer RA, Hahn EF, Fishman J. Naloxone, a specific opioid antagonist, reverses chronic idiopathic constipation. *Lancet* 1983;1:261-262.

86. Fotherby KJ, Hunter JO. Idiopathic slow-transit constipation: Whole gut transit times, measured by a new simplified method, are not shortened by opioid antagonists. *Aliment Pharmacol Ther* 1987;1:331-338.

87. Porter AJ, Wattchow DA, Hunter A, Costa M. Abnormalities of nerve fibers in the circular muscle of patients with slow transit constipation. *Int J Colorectal Dis* 1998;13:208-216.

88. Hoyle CHV, Kamm MA, Burnstock G, Lennard-Jones JE. Reduced activity of enkephalins in the colon of patients with idiopathic constipation (Abstract). *Gut* 1989;30:A709.

89. Dolk A, Broden G, Holmstrom B, Johansson C, Schultzberg M. Slow transit chronic constipation (Arbuthnot Lane's disease). An immunohistochemical study of neuropeptide-containing nerves in resected specimens from the large bowel. *Int J Colorectal Dis* 1990;5:181-187.

90. Koch TR, Carney JA, Go L, Go VL. Idiopathic chronic constipation is associated with decreased colonic vasoactive intestinal peptide. *Gastroenterology* 1988;94:300-310.

91. Lembo T, Naliboff BD, Matin K, Munakata J, Parker RA, Gracely RH, Mayer EA. Irritable bowel syndrome patients show altered sensitivity to exogenous opioids. *Pain* 2000;87:137-147.

92. Spiller R. Pharmacotherapy: Non-serotonergic mechanisms. *Gut* 2002;51 Suppl 1:i87-i90.

93. Hawkes ND, Rhodes J, Evans BK, Rhodes P, Hawthorne AB, Thomas GA. Naloxone treatment for irritable bowel syndrome—A randomized controlled trial with an oral formulation. *Aliment Pharmacol Ther* 2002;16:1649-1654.

Chapter 3

Opioid-Induced Immunosuppression

Gang Wei
Jonathan Moss
Chun-Su Yuan

Opioid medications are widely used clinically for relieving pain and as antidiarrheal and antitussives. Opioid agonists consist of a group of natural, semisynthetic, or synthetic compounds acting on a series of receptors, such as μ, κ, and δ receptors (discussed in Chapters 1 and 2). Concomitant with the ability to relieve pain, these drugs can have adverse effects. Side effects of opioid treatment include nausea, vomiting, constipation, respiratory suppression, fatigue, sweating, difficult micturition, psychomimetic disturbance, and dependence. Another less well-understood adverse effect of opioids is immunosuppression. This immunosuppression may also negatively affect the extent of opioid bowel dysfunction, mainly due to causing deterioration of body function in general.

Although opioid-induced immunosuppression is well described as a laboratory phenomenon in numerous animal experiments and clinical studies,[1] its overall importance as an adverse effect of opioid use has not been fully appreciated by physicians. The exact mechanisms of action of opioid effects on immunomodulation are incompletely understood, but several studies suggested that these immunomodulatory effects may be mediated via mechanisms different from those responsible for analgesia.

The introduction of an antagonist is a traditional element in the pharmacological proof of the receptor. Naloxone, naltrexone, and nalmefene are clinically prescribed opioid antagonists. These nonselective opioid receptor antagonists block both central analgesia and adverse effects of opioid medications, and therefore cannot discriminate between the analgesic and immunological effects. The recent development of peripheral opioid antagonists may permit greater understanding of the mechanisms of immunosuppression and be therapeutically relevant. Selective opioid antagonists have a potential for blocking undesired side effects of opioids, predominantly mediated by receptors peripherally located, while preserving the beneficial analgesic effect.[2,3] This chapter discusses possible sites of action of opioid-induced immunosuppression. If peripheral mechanisms do indeed play a significant role in opioid-induced immunosuppression, peripheral opioid antagonists may have a therapeutic role in clinical medicine.

STUDIES OF OPIOID-INDUCED IMMUNOSUPPRESSION

Animal and human studies have shown that opioids have profound effects on the immune system, a drug-induced immunological compromise. Increased rates of infection in animals treated with opioids,[4-6] as well as among heroin addicts,[7-9] have been demonstrated. Narcotic addicts are reported to have a markedly increased incidence of viral hepatitis, bacterial pneumonias, endocarditis, tuberculosis, and soft tissue and centeral nervous system (CNS) infections,[7,8,10,11] although confounding variables such as nutrition and access to care may make such correlations inexact.

Several studies in healthy normal individuals exposed to opioids have demonstrated the effect of opioids on immunomodulatory function.[12,13] Hamra and Yaksh observed that morphine inhibited lymphocyte proliferation, decreased splenic lymphocyte number, and altered phenotypic expression of cell surface markers.[14] Perhaps more important, chronically exposed individuals show a series of changes in their ability to respond to immunological challenges. Narcotic addicts and patients and animals receiving opioids exhibit abnormalities in many immunological parameters, including decreased natural killer (NK) cell cytolytic activity, blood lymphocyte proliferation responses to mitogen, and alterations in more complex immune responses including antibody-dependent cell-mediated cytotoxicity[15-17] and antibody production.[18-20] Opioids also have suppressive effects on hematopoietic cell development, resulting in atrophy of both the thymus and the spleen,[21-23] and reduced numbers of macrophages and B-cells in the murine spleen.[24]

Bayer et al. showed in vivo inhibition of lymphocyte proliferation by morphine, and this inhibition was completely antagonized by naltrexone pretreatment, suggesting involvement of opioid receptors.[25] In a well-known study, Yeager et al. observed that intravenous (iv) morphine inhibited NK cell cytotoxicity in volunteers.[26] However, a subsequent study in healthy subjects after fentanyl administration yielded a different conclusion.[27] These divergent results led to question whether the response to morphine is compound specific or a treatment regimen can be generalized to other opioids.

A recent observation greatly provides a possible mechanism for opioid-induced immunosuppression. Apoptosis (cell death) of immune cells is accelerated by directly inducing Fas (a death receptor) expression.[28] In a subsequent study of cells exposed to clinically relevant opioid doses, Yin et al. observed that stress modulated the immune system through CD95 (APO-1/Fas)-medicated apoptosis dependent on endogenous opioids. These investigators showed that chronically stressed mice exhibited a significant reduction in splenocytes, a process likely mediated by apoptosis, and an increase in CD95 expression. These stress-induced changes in lymphocyte number and CD95 expression could be blocked by naloxone or naltrexone.[29] In addition, the reduction of splenocytes they observed seems to be independent of the hypothalamic-pituitary-adrenal axis, since both adrenaletomized and sham-operated mice exhibited similar response to chronic stress.

The immunosuppressive characteristics of opioids have come into greater focus with the increase in patients with AIDS. A large number of HIV-1 infected individuals are drug abusers[30], and data show a correlation between drug abuse and HIV infection.[31,32] Morphine promotes the growth of HIV-1 in human peripheral blood mononuclear cell cultures.[33-34] Although the mechanism of increased HIV load in addicts is unclear, a recent study suggests a direct effect of opioids on CCR5 (a chemokine receptor that HIV uses as a coreceptor to gain entry in macrophages) turnover. Li et al. demonstrated that methadone in clinically relevant doses significantly enhanced HIV infection of macrophages with the up-regulation of expression of CCR5, a primary coreceptor for macrophage-tropic HIV entry into macrophages.[35] The relationship between opioid binding and CCR5 regulation remains to be further elucidated.

IS OPIOID-INDUCED IMMUNOSUPPRESSION
CENTRALLY MEDIATED?

Although a peripheral effect of opioids on lymphocyte regulation and HIV uptake is likely, evidence suggests that some elements of opioid-induced immunosupression may be centrally mediated. An early study in rats demonstrated that a very low dose of morphine (20 or 40 μg) injected into the lateral ventricle suppressed NK cell activity, and this effect was blocked by naltrexone, a nonselective opioid antagonist.[36] Hernandez et al. further examined whether the immunosuppressive effect of morphine is mediated by opioid receptors located at either peripheral or central sites.[37] First, the effects of systemic morphine administration on analgesia, mitogen-stimulated lymphocyte proliferation, and corticosterone secretion were compared to those observed after the systemic administration of N-methyl-morphine, a morphine analog that does not cross the blood-brain barrier. In contrast to morphine, N-methyl-morphine (20 mg·kg^{-1}) did not show any effect on lymphocyte proliferation, plasma corticosterone concentrations, or analgesic responses. Second, the effects of morphine and N-methyl-morphine after central administration were compared. With the microinjection of either morphine or N-methyl-morphine into the third ventricle, blood lymphocyte responses were inhibited by 70 percent; plasma corticosterone concentrations were significantly elevated; and maximal analgesic responses were present at the same time. Interestingly, a dissociation of immunosuppressive effects with antinociceptive action was noted when morphine was injected into the anterior hypothalamus. Blood lymphocyte proliferation decreased 50 percent, without an analgesic effect or a significant increase in plasma corticosterone.

Several studies have attempted to identify the specific brain regions involved in opioid-induced immunoregulation.[38-39] The periaqueductal gray matter (PAG) serves a variety of diverse autonomic functions and appears to be a candidate site for opioid action in the induction of immunosuppression. The PAG has been identified as a site of morphine-mediated naltrexone-sensitive suppression of rat splenic NK cell activity.[39] Opioid receptors and endogenous opioid peptides are present in the PAG, and endogenous opioids are released in the PAG during stress.[40] Further, microinjections of morphine into the

PAG specifically result in a rapid suppression of NK cell activity, and prior systemic administration of naltrexone can block NK cell suppression. These findings demonstrate that opioid-induced suppression of NK cell function is mediated at least in part through opioid receptors in the PAG.[39]

The immunosuppressive effects of acute morphine administration have been located to μ opioid receptors in the mesencephalon PAG region.[39-41] Gomez-Flores and Weber investigated morphine's and buprenorphine's abilities in influencing immune function after central administration.[38] Acute administration of morphine showed significant decreases in NK cell cytotoxic activity, T lymphocyte proliferative responses to various mitogens, and macrophages' functions, which were associated with high glucocorticoid and catecholamine levels. However, buprenorphine, a partial opioid agonist, did not alter immune function and also failed to increase the peripheral production of plasma glucocorticoids and catecholamines. Morphine has been suggested to induce immunosuppression by mainly interacting with μ_2 opioid receptors,[42] while buprenorphine has been observed to bind to μ_1 and κ opioid receptors.[43-44]

Although immune cells express μ, δ, and κ receptors which are functionally coupled with signal transductional mechanisms,[45] evidence suggests central μ receptors play a role in immunomodulation, but neither δ nor κ opioid receptors are involved.[46-47] Schneider and Lysle[48] showed that intracerebroventricular administration of the m-selective opioid agonist [D-Ala2, N-MePhe4, Gly5-ol] enkephalin (AMGO) to rats increased splenocytes' production of nitric oxide, a substance which may be linked to central immunomodulation, and this DAMGO's effect was blocked by prior methylnaltrexone injection. In contrast, intracerebroventricular administration of the κ selective agonist U69,593 and the δ selective agonist [D-Pen2, D-Pen5] enkephalin (DPDPE) had no significant effect on the production of nitric oxide. Nowak et al. also demonstrated that injection of SNC 80, a nonpeptidic δ-opioid receptor-selective agonist, in rats did not affect splenic NK cell activity.[49] The notion that μ opioid receptors within the CNS are responsible for the effect on immune function was further supported by another animal study, in which comparable results were obtained after administration of μ, κ, and δ agonists to the ventricle.[46] Involvement of central μ receptors in immunomosuppression has also been observed in a recent study,[50] in which rats received remifentanil, a pure μ receptor agonist with a half-life of only several minutes. The animals showed immunosuppressive effects similar to other μ receptor agonists.

While the immunological effects of opioids may be at least in part initiated centrally, there is evidence of a coordinated central and peripheral effect in mediating immunosuppression. Two possible pathways that have been implicated in the mediation of the immunomodulatory effects of morphine are (1) the hypothalamic-pituitary-adrenal (HPA) axis and (2) the sympathetic nervous system. In this respect, signals from the CNS to the immune system are relayed primarily through the HPA axis or via sympathetic innervation of lymphoid organs. Thus, opioid action in the HPA axis through hypothalamic efferents or enhanced opioid activity in the PAG could cause an increase in peripheral sympathetic output,[51] either of which could have an effect on NK cell activity.[52] The activation of the HPA axis results in the downstream production of glucocorticoids, which are immunosuppressives.[53-54] On the other hand, activation of the sympathetic nervous system elicits the release of biologic amines which have been demonstrated to suppress the immune system[55] by direct and secondary action on lymphocytes. While trying to reconcile these two hypotheses, it has been suggested that acute administration of opioids primarily alters peripheral immune function through the sympathetic nervous system, while chronic exposure to such compounds affects the immune system by activation of the HPA axis.[47]

Investigators have utilized methylnaltrexone, a quaternary form of naltrexone that does not cross the brain-blood barrier, to separate central from peripheral effects. The compound was able to antagonize most of the immune alterations produced by systemic morphine injection when administered intracerebroventricularly, but failed to do so when administered subcutaneously in rats.[56-58] At first glance this might be taken as proof that the CNS opioid receptors play an important role in the immune alterations by morphine. However, relatively low doses of methylnaltrexone were used in their in vivo studies, and receptor binding data showed that opioid receptor affinity of methylnaltrexone is approximately 20 to 100 times less compared to that of naltrexone.[59-60] Further, in addition, small animals, such as rats and mice, demethylated methylnaltrexone over time as shown by the exhalation of $^{14}CO_2$ after administration of (^{14}C-methyl) naltrexone methyl bromide.[2]

IS OPIOID-INDUCED IMMUNOSUPPRESSION PERIPHERALLY MEDIATED?

Although there is evidence for centrally mediated opioid immuno-suppression, there are also studies demonstrating that immunological dysfunction is mediated directly by opioid receptors located on immune cells. Morphine was found to decrease phagocytic activity of macrophages in a concentration-dependent manner, and naltrexone completely blocked the effects of morphine both in vivo and in vitro paradigms.[61] Bone marrow cells from mice implanted with morphine pellets showed a significant decrease in their developing capacity from macrophage precursors into viable colonies in response to macrophage colony stimulating factor, and this effect was inhibited by naltrexone.[62] Also, addition of morphine or β endorphin to precursor cells of macrophages had similar effect, showing that morphine acted directly on the precursor cells. Bayer et al.[25] observed that morphine inhibited concanavalin A–induced proliferation of both whole blood and splenic lymphocytes, although this inhibitory effect on the proliferation of lymphocytes could not be attenuated by co-incubation with naltrexone. The recent development of μ opioid receptor knockout mice has failed to reveal the mechanism of opioid-induced immmosuppression. Roy et al.[63] demonstrated that morphine reduction of splenic and thymic cell number and mitogen-induced proliferation were unaffected in the μ opioid knockout mice, suggesting non μ opioid or nonopioid actions on binding site of immune cells.

Thomas et al. [64] reported that, after in vitro exposure to morphine and its metabolites, a number of immunosuppressive effects were observed in immune cells obtained from both laboratory animals and humans. Taub et al.[65] and Eisenstein et al.[66] showed that morphine and κ agonists (U50,488H and U69,593) inhibited antibody formation when added to mouse spleen cells in vitro, indicating that the effects of these compounds act directly on immune cells. Furthermore, in vitro application of DAMGO, DPDPE, or U69,593 to splenocyte cultures did not significantly alter the production of nitric oxide by splenocytes. Thus, it seems unlikely that the suppression observed is mediated via the HPA axis or sympathetic nervous system. Guan et al. examined the effect of U50,488H, when added in vitro to T cell- or macrophage-enriched fractions of normal mouse spleens and found that the compound inhibited activity of both of these cell types.[67] In addition, the suppressive effects of a κ-agonist were observed on plaque-forming cell antibody response in rats, whether given in vivo or in vitro.[68] In contrast, evidence shows that by the inhibition of the chemokine receptor CXCR4 expression, κ-agonist has suppressive effect on HIV-1 entry into CD4+ lymphocytes with time-dependent[69] and concentration-response manner.[70]

Altogether, while κ receptors may be responsible for peripherally mediated immunosuppression, the contribution from μ or δ receptors remains to be determined. At the present, two peripheral opioid antagonists, methylnaltrexone and ADL 8-2698 (alvimopan), are under clinical investigation.[2,71] However, unlike methylnatrexone, alvimopan is only available in oral formulation without gut absorption. To the extent that the immunosuppression is peripherally mediated, parenterally administered peripheral opioid antagonists, such as methylnaltrexone,[72] may have a therapeutic role in reducing or eliminating opioid immunosuppressive action without affecting analgesia.

SUMMARY AND FUTURE WORK

In addition to their widespread illicit use and their role in addiction, opioid medications are a mainstay of perioperative care and chronic pain management. It has become increasingly clear that many of the side effects of opioids can be limiting factors of opioid use. While the focus has been on clinically apparent side effects, such as respiratory suppression and constipation, immunosuppression may be even more problematic, particularly in targeted populations. Evidence indicates that a close relationship exists between the use of opioids and immunological responses and infections, including HIV. The maintenance of immunological competence in the surgical population is a special challenge for medical professionals. Although numerous studies have demonstrated the effects of opioids to be suppressive on phagocytic, NK, B, and T cells in both animals and humans, the problem is complex as the site of action of opioids' immunosuppressive effects remains controversial. The weight of evidence suggests that opioids can act within the CNS and logically alter immunological competency. Understanding the immunosuppressive effect of opioids is complicated by differences among organ systems, specific testing compounds, the precise experimental conditions, and differences of effect among species. The precise mechanism of opioid effects on immunomodulation is incompletely understood. Important new tools may permit a more complete understanding of the anatomic and pharmacological targets of opioids on the immune system. In addition, the effect of such importance merits further explanations. If peripherally mediated immunosuppressive effects play a significant role in opioid-induced immunosuppression, the use of selective peripheral opioid antagonists in humans could potentially attenuate opioid-induced immunosuppression while preserving beneficial analgesic effect.

NOTES

1. Eisenstein TK, Hilburger ME. Opioid modulation of immune responses: Effects on phagocyte and lymphoid cell populations. *J Neuroimmunol* 1998;15;83: 36-44.

2. Yuan CS, Foss JF. Methylnaltrexone: Investigation of clinical applications. *Drug Dev Res* 2000;50:133-141.

3. Yuan CS, Foss JF, O'Connor M, Osinski J, Karrison T, Moss J, Roizen MF. Methylnaltrexone for reversal of constipation due to chronic methadone use: A randomized, controlled trial. *JAMA* 2000;283:367-372.

4. Tubaro E, Borelli G, Croce C. Effect of morphine on resistance to infection. *J Infect Dis* 1983;148:656-666.

5. Risdahl JM, Peterson PK, Chao CC, Pijoan C, Molitor TW. Effects of morphine dependence on the pathogenesis of swine herpesvirus infection. *J Infect Dis* 1993;167:1281-1287.

6. Risdahl JM, Khanna KV, Peterson KW, Molitor TW. Opioids and infections. *J Neuroimmunol* 1998;83:4-18.

7. Hussey HH, Katz S. Infections resulting from narcotic addiction. *Am J Med* 1950;9:186-193.

8. Haverkos HW, Lange WR. Serious infections other than human immunodeficiency virus among intravenous drug abusers. *J Infect Dis* 1990;161:894-912.

9. Quinn TC. The epidemiology of the acquired immunodeficiency syndrome in the 1990's. *Emerg Med Clin North Am* 1995;13:1-25.

10. Louria DB, Hensle T, Rose J. The major medical complications of heroin addiction. *Ann Int Med* 1967;67:1-22.

11. Reichman LB, Felton CP, Edsall JR. Drug dependence, a possible new risk factor for tuberculosis disease. *Arch Intern Med* 1979;139:337-339.

12. Crone LL, Conly JM, Clark KM, Chrichlow AC, Wardell GC, Zbitnew A, Rea LM, Cronk SL, Anderson CM, Tan LK, Albritton WL. Recurrent herpes simplex virus labialis and the use of epidural morphine in obstetric patients. *Anesth Analg* 1988;67:318-323.

13. Biagini RE, Henningsen GM, Klincewicz SL. Immunological analysis of peripheral leukocytes from workers at an ethical narcotics manufacturing facility. *Arch Environ Health* 1995;50(1):7-12.

14. Hamra JG, Yaksh TL. Equianalgesic doses of subcutaneous but not intrathecal morphine alter phenotypic expression of cell surface markers and mitogen-induced proliferation in rat lymphocytes. *Anesthesiology* 1996;85(2):355-365.

15. Layon J, Idris A, Warzynski M, Sherer R, Brauner D, Patch O, McCulley D, Orris P. Altered T-lymphocyte subsets in hospitalized intravenous drug abusers. *Arch Intern Med* 1984;144:1376-1380.

16. Nair MPN, Laing TJ, Schwartz SA. Decreased natural and antibody-dependent cellular cytotoxic activities in intravenous drug abusers. *Clin Immunol Immunopathol* 1986;38:68-78.

17. Molitor TW, Morilla A, Risdahl JM. Chronic morphine administration impairs cell-mediated immune responses in swine. *J Pharmacol Exp Ther* 1991;260:581-586.

18. Brown SM, Stimmel B, Taub RN, Kochwa S, Rosenfield RE. Immunological dysfunction in heroin addicts. *Arch Intern Med* 1974;134:1001-1006.

19. Morgan EL. Regulation of human B lymphocyte activation by opioid peptide hormones. Inhibition of IgG production by opioid receptor class (mu-, kappa-, and delta-) selective agonists. *J Neuroimmunol* 1996;65(1):21-30.

20. Palm S, Lehzen S, Mignat C, Steinmann J, Leimenstoll G, Maier C. Does prolonged oral treatment with sustained-release morphine tablets influence immune function? *Anesth Analg* 1998;86(1):166-172.

21. Bryant H, Bernton E, Holaday J. Immunosupressive effects of chronic morphine treatment in mice. *Life Sci* 1987;41:1731-1738.

22. Hilburger ME, Adler MW, Rogers TJ, Eisenstein TK. Morphine alters macrophage and lymphocyte populations in the spleen and peritoneal cavity. *J Neuroimmunol* 1997;80:106-114.

23. Freier DO, Fuchs BA. Morphine-induced alterations in thymocyte subpopulations of B6C3F1 mice. *J Pharmacol Exp Ther* 1993;265:81-88.

24. Singhal P, Sharma P, Kapasi A. Morphine enhances macrophage apoptosis. *J Immunol* 1998;160:1886-1893.

25. Bayer BM, Gastonguay MR, Hernandez MC. Distinction between the in vitro and in vivo inhibitory effects of morphine on lymphocyte proliferation based on agonist sensitivity and naltrexone reversibility. *Immunopharmacology* 1992;23(2):117-124.

26. Yeager MP, Colacchio TA, Yu CT. Morphine inhibits spontaneous and cytokine-enhanced natural killer cell cytotoxicity in volunteers. *Anesthesiology* 1995;83:500-508.

27. Yeager MP, Procopio MA, DeLeo JA, Arruda JL, Hildebrandt L, Howell AL. Intravenous fentanyl increases natural killer cell cytotoxicity and circulating CD16(+) lymphocytes in humans. *Anesth Analg* 2002;94:94-99.

28. Yin D, Mufson RA, Wang R, Shi YF. Fas-mediated cell death promoted by opioids. *Nature* 1999;397(6716):218.

29. Yin D, Tuthill D, Mufson RA, Shi Y. Chronic restraint stress promotes lymphocyte apoptosis by modulating CD95 expression. *J Exp Med* 2000;191:1423-1428.

30. Swan N. CDC report highlights link between drug abuse and spread of HIV *NIDA Notes* 1997;12(2). Available at: <http://www.drugabuse.gov/NIDA_Notes/NNVol12N2/CDCReports.html>.

31. Donahoe RM, Falek A. Neuroimmunomodulation by opiates and other drugs of abuse: Relationship to HIV infection and AIDS. *Adv Biochem Psychopharmacol* 1988;44:145-158.

32. Centers for Disease Control and Prevention. *HIV/AIDS surveillance report,* 1995;7(2). Available at: <http://www.aegis.org/pubs/surveil/1995/HIVSUR72.html>.

33. Peterson PK, Gekker G, Lokensgard JR, Bidlack JM, Chang CA, X. Fang X, Portoghese PS. κ-Opioid receptor agonist suppression of HIV-1 expression in CD4+ lymphocytes. *Biochem Pharmacol* 2001;61:1145-1151.

34. Chao CC, Gekker G, Hu S. Upregulation of HIV-1 expression in cocultures of chronically infected promonocytes and human brain cells by dynorphin. *Biochem Pharmacol* 1995;50:715-722.

35. Li Y, Wang X, Tian S, Guo CJ, Douglas SD, Ho WZ. Methadone enhances human immunodeficiency virus infection of human immune cells. *J Infect Dis* 2002;185(1):118-122.

36. Shavit Y, Depaulis A, Martin FC, Terman GW, Pechnick RN, Zane CJ, Gale RP, Liebeskind JC. Involvement of brain opioid receptors in the immune-suppressive effect of morphine. *Proc Natl Acad Sci* 1986;83:7114-7117.

37. Hernandez MC, Flores LR, Bayer BM. Immunosuppression by morphine is mediated by central pathways. *J Pharmacol Exp Ther* 1993;267:336-341.

38. Gomez-Flores R, Weber RJ. Differential effects of buprenorphine and morphine on immune and neuroendocrine functions following acute administration in the rat mesencephalon periaqueductal gray. *Immunopharmacology* 2000;48(2): 145-156.

39. Weber RJ, Pert A. The periaqueductal gray matter mediates opioid-induced immunosuppression. *Science* 1989;245;188-190.

40. Seeger TF, Sforzo GA, Pert CB, Pert A. In vivo autoradiography: Visualization of stress-induced changes in opioid receptor occupancy in the rat brain. *Brain Res* 1984;305(2):303-311.

41. Lysle DT, Hoffman KE, Dykstra LA. Evidence for the involvement of the caudal region of the periaqueductal gray in a subset of morphine-induced alterations of immune status. *J Pharmacol Exp Ther* 1996;277(3):1533-1540.

42. Carr DJ, Gebhardt BM, Paul D. Alpha adrenergic and mu-2 opioid receptors are involved in morphine-induced suppression of splenocyte natural killer activity. *J Pharmacol Exp Ther* 1993;264(3):1179-1186.

43. Kamei J, Sodeyama M, Tsuda M, Suzuki T, Nagase H. Antinociceptive effect of buprenorphine in mu1-opioid receptor deficient CXBK mice. *Life Sci* 1997; 60(22):333-337.

44. Pick CG, Peter Y, Schreiber S, Weizman R. Pharmacological characterization of buprenorphine, a mixed agonist-antagonist with kappa 3 analgesia. *Brain Res* 1997;744(1):41-46.

45. Carr DJ, Rogers TJ, Weber RJ. The relevance of opioids and opioid receptors on immunocompetence and immune homeostasis. *Proc Soc Exp Biol Med* 1996; 213:248-257.

46. Nelson CJ, Schneider GM, Lysle DT. Involvement of central μ- but not δ- or κ-opioid receptors in immunomodulatoin. *Brain Behavor Immunity* 2000;14:170-184.

47. Mellon RD, Bayer BM. Role of central opioid receptor subtypes in morphine-induced alterations in peripheral lymphocyte activity. *Brain Res* 1998; 789(1):56-67.

48. Schneider GM, Lysle DT. Role of central mu-opioid receptors in the modulation of nitric oxide production by splenocytes. *J Neuroimmunol* 1998;89:150-159.

49. Nowak JE, Gomez-Flores R, Calderon SN, Rice KC, Weber RJ. Rat natural killer cell, T cell and macrophage functions after intracerebroventricular injection of SNC 80. *J Pharmacol Exp Ther* 1998;286(2):931-937.

50. Sacerdote P, Gaspani L, Rossoni G, Panerai AE, Bianchi M. Effect of the opioid remifentanil on cellular immune response in the rat. *Int Immunopharmacol* 2001;1:713-719.

51. Blalock JE. The immune system as a sensory organ. *J Immunol* 1984; 132(3):1067-1070.

52. Felten DL, Felten SY, Carlson SL, Olschowka JA, Livnat S. Noradrenergic and peptidergic innervation of lymphoid tissue. *J Immunol* 1985;135(2 Suppl): 755s-765s.

53. Pruett SB, Han YC, Fuchs BA. Morphine suppresses primary humoral immune responses by a predominantly indirect mechanism. *J Pharmacol Exp Ther* 1992;262:923-928.

54. Freier DO, Fuchs BA. A mechanism of action for morphine-induced immunosuppression: Corticosterone mediates morphine-induced suppression of natural killer cell activity. *J Pharmacol Exp Ther* 1994;270(3):1127-1133.

55. Fecho K, Maslonek KA, Dykstra LA, Lysle DT. Evidence for sympathetic and adrenal involvement in the immunomodulatory effects of acute morphine treatment in rats. *J Pharmacol Exp Ther* 1996;277(2):633-645.

56. Lysle DT, Luecken LJ, Maslonek KA. Modulation of immune status by a conditioned aversive stimulus: Evidence for the involvement of endogenous opioids. *Brain Behav Immun* 1992;6(2):179-188.

57. Lysle DT, Coussons-Read ME. Mechanisms of conditioned immunomodulation. *Int J Immunopharmacol* 1995;17(8):641-647.

58. Fecho K, Maslonek KA, Dykstra LA, Lysle DT. Assessment of the involvement of central nervous system and peripheral opioid receptors in the immunomodulatory effects of acute morphine treatment in rats. *J Pharmacol Exp Ther* 1996;276(2):626-636.

59. Yuan CS, Foss JF, Moss J. Effects of methylnaltrexone on morphine-induced inhibition of contraction in isolated guinea-pig ileum and human intestine. *Eur J Pharmacol* 1995;276:107-111.

60. Yuan CS, Foss JF. Gastric effects of methylnaltrexone on mu, kappa and delta opioid agonists induced brainstem unitary responses. *Neuropharmacology* 1999; 38:425-432.

61. Rojavin M, Szabo I, Bussiere J. Morphine treatment in vitro or in vivo decreases phagocytic functions of murine macrophages. *Life Sci* 1993;53:997-1006.

62. Roy S, Ramakrishnan S, Loh HH, Lee NM. Chronic morphine treatment selectively suppresses macrophage colony formation in bone marrow. *Eur J Pharmacol* 1991;195:359-363.

63. Roy S, Barke RA, Loh HH. MU-opioid receptor-knockout mice: Role of mu-opioid receptor in morphine mediated immune functions. *Brain Res Mol Brain Res* 1998;61:190-194.

64. Thomas PT, Bhargava HN, House RV. Immunomodulatory effects of in vitro exposure to morphine and its metabolites. *Pharmacology* 1995;50:51-62.

65. Taub DD, Eisenstein TK, Geller EB, Adler MW, Rogers TJ. Immunomodulatory activity of μ- and κ-selective opioid agonists. *Proc Natl Acad Sci* 1991;88:360-364.

66. Eisenstein TK, Meissler Jr. JJ, Rogers TJ, Geller EB, Adler MW. Mouse strain differences in immunosuppression by opioids in vitro. *J Pharmacol Exp Ther* 1995;275:1484-1489.

67. Guan L, Townsend R, Eisenstein TK, Adler MW, Rogers TJ. Both T cells and macrophages are targets of κ-opioid-induced immunosuppression. *Brain Behav Immun* 1994;8:229-240.

68. Radulovic J, Miljevic C, Djergovic D, Vujic V, Antic J, von Horsten S, Jankovic BD. Opioid receptor-mediated suppression of humoral immune response in vivo and in vitro: Involvement of κ-opioid receptors. *J Neuroimmunol* 1995; 57:55-62.

69. Peterson PK, Gekker G, Lokensgard JR, Bidlack JM, Chang AC, Fang X, Portoghese PS. Kappa-opioid receptor agonist suppression of HIV-1 expression in CD4+ lymphocytes. *Biochem Pharmacol* 2001;61(9):1145-1151.

70. Lokensgard JR, Gekker G, Peterson PK. κ-Opioid receptor agonist inhibition of HIV-1 envelope glycoprotein-mediated membrane fusion and CXCR4 expression on CD4+ lymphocytes. *Biochem Pharmacol* 2002;63(6):1037-1041.

71. Taguchi A, Sharma N, Saleem RM, Sessler DI, Carpenter RL, Seyedsadr M, Kurz A. Selective postoperative inhibition of gastrointestinal opioid receptors. *N Engl J Med* 2001;345:935-940.

72. Moss J, Yuan CS. Selective postoperative inhibition of gastrointestinal opioid receptors. *N Engl J Med* 2002;346:455.

SECTION II:
CLINICAL STATES

Chapter 4

The Epidemiology of Opioid Bowel Dysfunction

Ysmael Yap
Marco Pappagallo

INTRODUCTION

Opioids are widely employed in the control of acute and chronic pain due to malignant and nonmalignant diseases. The World Health Organization (WHO) guidelines for the management of moderate to severe pain recommend the use of opioid analgesics.[1] Opioids are currently the mainstay treatment for patients with chronic cancer pain and may represent the major source of relief for many patients with moderate to severe nonmalignant pain.[2]

Even though the therapeutic success of opioid therapy in the control of pain is well established, opioids can also cause a variety of adverse effects, including respiratory depression, sedation, nausea, vomiting, pruritus, miosis, as well as constipation. Unlike other side effects, tolerance to constipation may develop very slowly or not at all with prolonged opioid use.[3]

Opioid receptors are found not only in the brain and spinal cord but also in peripheral nerves and in the myoneuroenteric plexus of the intestinal wall. The opioid receptors mu (μ), delta (δ), and kappa (κ) can be activated by both endogenous (endorphins, enkephalins, and dynorphins) and exogenous (e.g., morphine, oxycodone) opioid agonists.[4] In the central nervous system (CNS), the primary receptors

The authors thank the following staff members of the Department of Pain Medicine and Palliative Care at Beth Israel Medical Center, New York: Peter Homel, PhD, and Russell K Portenoy, MD, for his valuable suggestions.

involved in analgesia are the μ receptors.[4,5] In the periphery, activation of the μ receptors affects a variety of gastrointestinal (GI) functions, such as motility, secretion, and absorption (see Table 4.1).[6] Opioid-induced GI functional changes can be both centrally and peripherally mediated.[7]

GASTROINTESTINAL
ADVERSE EFFECTS OF OPIOIDS

Opioid therapy sometimes can be associated with a syndrome of very severe constipation and a poorly recognized condition known as opioid bowel dysfunction (OBD). OBD comprises a constellation of GI adverse events that may occur during short-term and long-term opioid use. OBD is characterized by

1. hard, dry stools;
2. straining;
3. incomplete evacuation;
4. bloating;
5. abdominal distention; and
6. increased gastric reflux.[2]

TABLE 4.1. Pharmacological effects of opioids on gastrointestinal functions: Opioid bowel dysfunction.

Pharmacologic action of opioids	Clinical effects
Decreased gastric motility and emptying	Increased gastroesophageal reflux
Inhibition of intestinal propulsion	Delayed adsorption of medications, incomplete evacuation, bloating, abdominal distension
Increased amplitude of nonpropulsive segmental contractions	Spasm, abdominal cramps, and pain
Constriction of sphincter of Oddi	Biliary colic, epigastric discomfort
Increased anal sphincter tone	Impaired ability to evacuate the bowel
Diminished gastric, biliary, pancreatic, and intestinal secretions	Hard, dry stool

Source: Adapted and revised from Reisine T, Pasternak G. Opioid analgesics and antagonists. In Hardman JG, Limbird LE, Gilman AG, (eds.), *Goodman & Gilman's The pharmacologic basis of therapeutics,* 9th edition. New York. Pergamon Press, 1996:521-555.

In severe cases of OBD, some patients choose to limit or discontinue opioid use in an effort to reduce the additional discomfort associated with OBD.[8,9] Persistent or unrecognized symptoms associated with OBD can negatively impact the patient's quality of life and lead to deterioration of functional status.[10,11]

Certain opioid-induced effects, such as decreased stomach emptying or inhibition of small and large intestinal motility, appear to correlate with specific clinical manifestations of OBD (Table 4.1).[12] At its worst, GI dysfunction can result in ileus, fecal impaction, and obstruction.[13,14] Among the different opioid derivatives, OBD seems to be more pronounced with codeine[15] and less with transdermal opioids (e.g., fentanyl).[16]

Constipation has no clear-cut definition. According to *Dorland's Medical Dictionary,* constipation is defined as infrequent or difficult evacuation of the feces.[17] As an operational definition, constipation can be defined by the arbitrary criterion of fewer than three satisfactory (i.e., full, complete) bowel movements per week.[2]

PREVALENCE IN THE GENERAL POPULATION

The prevalence of constipation in the U.S. general population showed a wide range of variation from an estimate of 2 to 28 percent.[18,19] The wide variation could be attributed to the problem of how constipation is defined.[20]

A study of the epidemiology of constipation in the general population in the United States in 1999 found that the overall prevalence of constipation in the U.S. population is 14.7 percent. Prevalence according to subtype was 4.6 percent for functional, 2.1 percent for irritable bowel syndrome (IBS), 4.6 percent for outlet obstruction (also known as anismus,[21] pelvic floor dyssynergia,[22] and obstructive defecation[23]), and 3.4 percent for IBS outlet (combination)-associated constipation.[19]

PREVALENCE IN THE OPIOID-TREATED POPULATION

Estimates vary as to the prevalence of constipation in patients treated with opioids, but all are much higher than the rate in the general population. In a prospective study of 1,635 cancer pain patients, 33 percent reported constipation.[24] Constipation-related symptoms increased significantly after initiation of morphine despite pretreatment with a prophylactic bowel regimen containing bisacodyl, a stimulant laxative, and lactulose.[25]

A survey of patients admitted to a Midwestern hospital oncology unit found that 97 percent of the 60 patients interviewed were satisfied with their level of pain control. At the same time, however, more than 95 percent of these patients cited constipation as a major side effect of their opioid regimen.[26] Similar results hold for patients with noncancer pain. One source reports a 41 percent incidence of constipation in morphine-treated patients.[27]

A detailed survey was conducted in Baltimore, Maryland, to evaluate the prevalence of constipation in a group of 76 opioid-treated patients.[28] These patients were treated for chronic nonmalignant pain and received at least 10 mg/day or more of oral morphine for 5 or more weeks. The opioid-treated group was compared with a U.S. population sample group involving 10,018 adults surveyed by telephone interview.[2]

The study comparing opioid-treated patients against random U.S. survey participants revealed that the former were five times more likely than the latter to be constipated (less than three complete bowel movements per week) (see Table 4.2), and were almost twice as likely to require treatment for constipation (80 versus 58 percent) while being less than half as likely to experience relief from laxative use (25 versus 55 percent). Compared to the U.S. survey population who tended to use bowel stimulants and fiber supplements, the opioid-treated patients were typically older (51 percent were older than 51 years versus 40 percent), Caucasian (87 versus 80 percent), less educated (21 versus 32 percent), and were more likely to be obese (57 percent had body mass indexes greater than 27.3 versus 32 percent).[2] The opioid-treated patients required more complicated treatment modalities including stool softeners, stimulant laxatives, lubricants, osmotic agents, and other medications with secondary or off-label laxative effects.[2]

TABLE 4.2. Survey results comparing bowel habits and constipation-related treatments: General U.S. versus opioid users.

Variable	U.S. survey sample (*n* = 10,018)	Opioid users (*n* = 76)
BMs*/week (median)	7.0	5.0
Complete BMs/week (median)	7.0	4.0
Incomplete BMs	8.8 %	36.1 %
Straining	8.9 %	40.0 %
Hard and lumpy stool	16.0 %	45.4 %
Patients with <3 complete BMs/week	7.6 %	40.3 %
Patients taking laxatives for constipation	55.0 %	80.0 %
Patients achieving desired result with laxatives half of the time	84.0 %	46.0 %

Source: Adapted and revised from Pappagallo M. Incidence, prevalence, and management of opioid bowel dysfunction. *Am J. Surg.* 2001;182(5A Suppl):11S-18S.
*BM = Bowel movement.

DISCUSSION

In summary, long-term opioid use for pain control resulted in greater bowel dysfunction, which was largely unresponsive to treatment with laxatives. Further investigations should be directed toward improving pharmacologic and nonpharmacologic preventive modalities for chronic opioid users.

Although not all patients on opioid therapy develop constipation, the majority are likely to complain of the symptom. It is important to rule out different coexisting morbidities that can produce constipation in patients requiring an opioid treatment regimen to control pain. Recognizing that constipation is one of the most common debilitating adverse effects in patient on opioid therapy, it is imperative to consider a bowel regimen at the start of the opioid treatment, especially in those patients who already have GI problems and are predisposed to constipation.

A proactive approach is also an important principle of pain management,[29] especially in the prevention of side effects. This includes preventive measures such as adequate fluid intake, appropriate diet (high fiber, natural roughage), exercises, providing an atmosphere of privacy, and convenience, which are all important aspects of bowel management. Although it is unlikely that taking these steps will be sufficient for preventing opioid-induced constipation in many patients,[29] they may at least lessen the seriousness and intensity of subsequent constipation onset. A combination of prophylaxis together with prompt medical intervention to alleviate the symptoms will result in better quality of life for the patient and possibly improved drug compliance.

NOTES

1. World Health Organization: *Cancer pain relief,* 2nd ed. Geneva: WHO; 1996.

2. Pappagallo M. Incidence, prevalence, and management of opioid bowel dysfunction. *Am J Surg* 2001;182(5A Suppl):11S-18S.

3. Pappagallo M. Aggressive pharmacologic treatment of pain. *Rheum Dis Clin North Am* 1999;25(1):193-213.

4. Friedman JD, Dello Buono FA. Opioid antagonists in the treatment of opioid-induced constipation and pruritus. *Ann Pharmacother* 2001;35(1):85-91.

5. Knowles CH, Martin JE. Slow transit constipation: A model of human gut dysmotility. Review of possible etiologies. *Neurogastroenterol Motil* 2000;12(2): 181-196.

6. De Luca A, Coupar IM. Insights into opioid action in the intestinal tract. *Pharmacol Ther* 1996; 69(2):103-115.

7. Manara L, Bianchetti A. The central and peripheral influences of opioids on gastrointestinal propulsion. *Ann Rev Pharmacol Toxicol* 1985;25:249-273.

8. Glare P, Lickiss JN. Unrecognized constipation in patients with advanced cancer: A recipe for therapeutic disaster. *J Pain Symptom Manage* 1992;7(6):369-371.

9. Whitecar PS, Jones AP, Clasen ME. Managing pain in dying patient. *Am Fam Physician* 2000;61(3):755-764.

10. Klepstad P, Kaasa S, Skauge M, et al. Pain intensity and side effects during titration of morphine to cancer patients using a fixed schedule dose escalation. *Acta Anaesthesiol Scand* 2000;44(6):656-664.

11. Fallon MT, Hanks GW. Morphine, constipation, and performance status in advance cancer patients. *Palliat Med* 1999;13(2):159-160.

12. Reisine T, Pasternak G. Opioid analgesics and antagonists. In Hardman JG, Limbird LE, Gilman AG, (eds.), *Goodman & Gilman's The pharmacologic basis of therapeutics,* 9th edition. New York: McGraw-Hill; 1996.

13. Levy MH. Pharmacologic management of cancer pain. *Semin Oncol* 1994; 21(6):718-739.

14. Lipman AG, Gauthier ME. Pharmacology of opioid drugs: Basic principles. In Portenoy RK, Bruera E (eds.), *Topics in palliative care,* Volume 1. New York, Oxford University Press; 1997:137-161.

15. Walsh TD. Prevention of opioid side effects. *J Pain Symptom Manage* 1990;5(6):362-367.

16. Ahmedzai S, Brook D. Transdermal fentanyl versus sustained-release oral morphine in cancer pain: preference, efficacy, and quality of life. The tts-fentanyl comparative trial group. *J Pain Symptom Manage* 1997;13(5):254-261.

17. Dorland WAN (ed.). *Dorland's illustrated medical dictionary.* 27th edition. Philadelphia: W.B. Saunders Company; 1988.

18. Sonnenberg A, Koch TR. Epidemiology of constipation in the United States. *Dis Colon Rectum* 1989;32:1-8.

19. Stewart WF, Liberman JN, Sandler RS, Woods MS, Stemhagen A, Chee E, Lipton RB, and Farup CE. Epidemiology of constipation (EPOC) study in the United States: Relation of clinical subtypes to sociodemographic features. *Am J Gastroenterol* 1999;94(12):3530-3540.

20. Rao SS. Constipation: Evaluation and treatment. *Gastroenterol Clin North Am* 2003;32(2):659-683.

21. Preston DM, Lennard-Jones J. Anismus in chronic constipation. *Dig Dis Sci* 1985;30:413-418.

22. Whitehead WE, Wald A, Diamant N, Enck P, Pemberton JH, Rad SS. Functional disorders of the anorectum. *Gut* 1999;45:55-59.

23. Rao SSC. Dyssynergic defecation: Disorders of the anorectum. *Gastroenterol Clin North Am* 2001;31:97-114.

24. Grond S, Zech D, Diefenbach C, Bischoff, A. Prevalence and pattern of symptoms in patients with cancer pain: A prospective evaluation of 1635 cancer patients referred to a pain clinic. *J Pain Symptom Manage* 1994;9(6):372-382.

25. Klepstad P, Borchgrevink PC, Kaasa S. Effects on cancer patients' health-related quality of life after the start of morphine therapy. *J Pain Symptom Manage* 2000;20(1):19-26.

26. Robinson CB, Fritch M, Hullett L, Petersen MA, Sikkema S, Theunink L, Timmer K. Development of a protocol to prevent opioid- induced constipation in patients with cancer: A research utilization project. *Clin J Oncol Nurs* 2000; 4(2):79-84.

27. Moulin DE, Iezzi A, Amireh R, Sharpe WK, Boyd D, Merskey H. Randomized trial of oral morphine for chronic non-cancer pain. *Lancet* 1996; 347(8995): 143-147.

28. Pappagallo M, Stewart W, Woods M. *Constipation symptoms in long-term users of opioid analgesic therapy.* Poster-Abstract. American Pain Society Annual Meeting, Fort Lauderdale, Florida, October 21-24, 1999.

29. Pasero C, Portenoy RK, McCaffery M. Opioid Analgesics. In McCaffery M, Pasero C (eds.), *Topics in pain clinical manual,* 2nd edition. St. Louis, MO: Mosby; 1999:162-299.

Chapter 5

Opioid Bowel Dysfunction in Palliative Care

Nigel P. Sykes

INTRODUCTION

The purpose of palliative care is the control of symptoms in patients with far-advanced incurable disease, often cancer, but with application to a wide range of other conditions. Its interest in bowel dysfunction is therefore in the symptoms that such dysfunction causes.

The most common and enduring of these symptoms is constipation. The other principal symptoms referable to opioid bowel dysfunction are nausea and vomiting, and this chapter considers the management of these two symptom groups. They are linked in what has been termed the *narcotic bowel syndrome* in which severe morphine-induced constipation mimics symptoms of intestinal obstruction.[1] Indeed, even in milder clinical situations nausea, and perhaps vomiting, can appear in association with constipation, and there is some early experimental evidence that constipation without the involvement of opioids can precipitate nausea.[2]

CONSTIPATION

At least half of all patients admitted to a palliative care unit complain of constipation, and the true figure is higher because others will already be receiving effective laxative treatment. Constipation has been found to cause a level of distress among palliative care patients rivalling that due to pain.[3-5]

The Problem of Definition

Because elsewhere in medicine constipation has an identity as a disease in its own right and because it has various measurable physical parameters that might be associated with it, attempts have been made to provide a quantitative definition of the condition. Most prominent among these are what are sometimes referred to as the "Rome criteria"[6] which state that constipation is present if two or more of the following symptoms have existed for more than three months:

- Straining at least 25 percent of the time
- Hard stools at least 25 percent of the time
- Incomplete evacuation at least 25 percent of the time
- Three or fewer bowel movements per week

These criteria are informed by epidemiological studies showing that 95[7] to 99 percent [8] of a healthy population defecates at least three times per week. They were designed for use in gastroenterological investigation of healthy patients presenting with chronic constipation. Unfortunately, it is common to meet people who think they are constipated while not meeting these criteria. Although they might agree that if they are constipated they pass stools less frequently or with difficulty, individuals may differ in the weight they give to these components of the definition or add new elements of their own.

For instance, in a survey of 93 cancer patients in the author's hospice unit, 46 said they were currently constipated. However, 68 had had a bowel movement either on the day of questioning or the day before. Only 32 reported frequent straining. Similarly, in a random sample of 531 family practice patients and 57 family physicians, over half of the patients defined constipation differently than the doctors did. The doctors used a frequency definition in accord with the Rome criteria, whereas 27 percent of the patients used a frequency definition of defecation every 2 days or less (i.e., an average of less than 3.5 bowel movements per week) and 25 percent defined constipation simply as hard stool.[9]

A group of patients who considered themselves constipated and who reported three or fewer bowel movements a week for at least six months completed stool diaries for four weeks. Fifty-one percent proved to have stool frequencies above this level (an average of six stools per week) and were deemed by the investigators not to be constipated. However, both groups of patients reported similar levels of difficulty in defecation, suggesting that this was a more important criterion of constipation for them than bowel movement frequency.[10]

Quite simply, people have their own personal definition of what it means to be constipated. This certainly tends to contain the components of the Rome definition, as 85 percent of the hospice cancer patients cited difficulty in passing stool as a symptom of constipation and 69 percent mentioned reduced frequency of defecation, but 45 percent also mentioned flatulence and abdominal bloating. There was no sense of a minimum time over which these symptoms had to persist.

The Rome criteria were intended to clarify the diagnosis of functional constipation in an essentially healthy population. When constipation is an accompaniment of illness, the time requirement, in particular, becomes less appropriate. No other symptom is approached in this way: relief is not offered for pain or breathlessness only after it has been endured for at least three months. In addition to the unnecessary suffering that this would cause, this period would be a substantial fraction of the life expectancy of many palliative care patients.

Etiology of Constipation

Constipation is a complaint of around 10 percent of the adult population in general, but nearer 20 percent of the elderly.[11] It has also repeatedly been reported to be more common in women.[12] The range of factors that potentially contribute to the occurrence of bowel dysfunction in palliative care is, of course, considerable and by no means confined to the use of opioid drugs (see Table 5.1). Physical illness in general is a risk factor for constipation: 63 percent of elderly people in hospitals have been found to be constipated, compared with 22 percent of the same age group living at home.[13]

Few medically ill patients have previously had persistent problems with constipation. Among the 93 palliative care patients with cancer previously mentioned, 78 reported that prior to illness they had rarely or never been constipated and only four had always been constipated. Now 50 of them experienced constipation all or most of the time (Sykes, unpublished observations). Indeed, constipation is more common in people terminally ill with cancer than in those dying of other

TABLE 5.1. Causes of constipation in palliative care.

Cause	Type	Contributing factor
Disease	Directly due to malignancy	Intestinal obstruction due to a tumor in the bowel wall or external compression by abdominal or pelvic tumor
		Damage to lumbosacral spinal cord, cauda equina, or pelvic plexus
		Hypercalcaemia
	Neurological disease	Damage to lumbosacral spinal cord, cauda equina, or pelvic plexus
	Due to secondary effects of disease	Inadequate food intake Low fiber diet Dehydration Weakness Inactivity Confusion Depression Autonomic impairment Institutional factors
Drugs	Opioids	
	Drugs with anticholinergic effects	Hyoscine Phenothiazines Tricyclic antidepressants Anti-Parkinsonian agents
	Antacids Diuretics Anticonvulsants Iron Antihypertensive agents Vincristine Cisplatin Ondansetron (predominant effect, but may also cause diarrhea)	Calcium and aluminum compounds
Concurrent disease	Diabetes Hypothyroidism Hypokalemia Hernia Diverticular disease Rectocele Anal fissure or stenosis Anterior mucosal prolapse Hemorrhoids Colitis	

causes.[14] Certain oncology treatments commonly have constipation as an adverse effect: up to 35 percent of those receiving vinca alkaloids have been reported to become constipated, as do 70 percent of patients given carboplatin.[15] Although it can also cause diarrhea, constipation is the most common side effect of ondansetron, often included as an antiemetic in chemotherapy regimes.

Constipation is also common across a range of neurological diseases.[16] A prevalence of 54 percent has been reported in multiple sclerosis[17] and 65 to 86 percent in advanced amyotrophic lateral sclerosis. Here, constipation may be due either to the neurological damage itself or may result nonspecifically from being chronically ill or from opioid or anticholinergic drugs used for symptom control.

The Contribution of Opioid Bowel Dysfunction to Constipation in Palliative Care

Opioid analgesics, specifically morphine, are probably the largest single identifiable constipating influence in patients who take them. Some 95 percent of oncology patients report constipation as the major side effect of their opioid analgesia.[18] Opioids appear to be responsible for around one-quarter of the constipation found in terminally ill patients. A study of 498 hospice patients found that 63 percent of those *not* taking morphine required laxatives, a figure similar to that found in the ill elderly, but 87 percent of those receiving morphine needed them and used a higher average dose.[19]

In this study oral laxative doses were compared with the mean of morphine doses within each quartile of morphine dose. The result was a histogram whose shape resembled that of the characteristic hyperbolic dose-response curve that might be expected from a drug-receptor interaction. Bowel movement frequency and the requirement for rectal laxatives did not vary significantly between morphine quartiles. It was inferred that the laxative doses were acting as an indirect measure of the degree of constipation and hence of the constipating effect of morphine at gut μ_2 receptors. The amount of laxative required even when the morphine intake was zero was an expression of the underlying constipation due to other illness-related factors. The scatter of morphine doses was quite considerable, which is unsurprising given the huge range of doses needed to achieve analgesia in apparently similar patients.

Measuring the Effect of Opioid Tolerance

The question arises as to whether tolerance to the constipating action of morphine might occur just as it can do to its pain-relieving action. The clinical impression is that if it occurs at all, such tolerance develops slowly and partially. Experimentally, μ_2 receptor mediated opioid actions such as delaying of intestinal transit show less development of tolerance than μ_1-mediated analgesia does.[20]

In the palliative care study previously mentioned,[19] patients followed for over two months ($n = 28$) did not differ significantly from the rest of the group in morphine or laxative consumption but did have higher stool frequencies and somewhat lower use of enemas and suppositories. Their median laxative dose rose over the review period but by much less than their median morphine dose.

In a smaller study, performed in a hospital palliative care population, twelve patients survived for six months. Among them were four who required no laxatives despite taking morphine, sometimes in substantial amounts.[21] It is not clear whether these four patients had never needed laxatives or whether they had at some point been able to give them up, i.e., whether they had become tolerant to the constipating effect of morphine or whether they lay at one extreme of the morphine dose-response curve for constipation.

It might be expected that palliative care patients with a longer prognosis would have milder constipation than those who are more ill: they will be eating and drinking more and they will be more mobile. Thus although it is possible that tolerance to the gut effects of morphine does occur, the phenomenon has yet to be quantified.

Comparing the Constipating Power of Opioids

As the range of alternative strong opioids to morphine has increased, there has been growing interest in the possibility that some may cause less constipation. Particular attention has been paid to fentanyl in its transdermal formulation. Several crossover trials have reported fentanyl to be less constipating than morphine, but a number have exhibited methodological flaws in relying on subjective assessments of constipation without measuring laxative intake. Also, different morphine:fentanyl dose conversion ratios have been used, making it unclear whether the fentanyl dose truly matches the potency of the morphine.

A recent trial of fentanyl and morphine has addressed most of these issues in using a relatively higher dose of fentanyl than some others, obtaining stool frequency and consistency data from patient diaries, and taking the as-required use of laxatives (which are detailed) as an outcome variable.[22] Over a 30-day study period laxative use was significantly ($p < 0.001$) less than during the preceding week when morphine was being used, without any change in bowel movement frequency.

Among other opioids, reduction in laxative use has been reported after changing from morphine to methadone, but to date only on a case history basis.[23] Oxycodone has not shown constipating effects significantly different from those of morphine[24] and neither has hydromorphone.[25] Tramadol lacks the sphincter contraction effects of morphine and is reported to be less constipating than either oxycodone or codeine.[26]

EVALUATION OF CONSTIPATION

History

A complaint of constipation needs to be clarified by a careful history. The prior pattern of defecation should be sought as a basis for comparison with the current frequency and difficulty of bowel movements. It should be established whether constipation predated the present illness, as this may justify wider investigations. Symptoms such as abdominal pain, bloating, flatulence, nausea, malaise, headache, and halitosis are associated by some patients with constipation, but these are nonspecific and most can occur also with diarrhea.

Constipation Assessment Tools

Objective Assessments

In the context of concurrent illness, the importance of constipation is as a symptom, and hence it is the patient's perspective that is most valid. However, the widely accepted Rome criteria[6] invite the measurement of objective outcomes, which are taken to be indicators of the severity of constipation. Whether they also reflect the impact of disordered bowel function upon the patient is much less clear.

In the palliative care setting invasive measurement of the parameters of bowel function is not possible or appropriate. However, an estimate of the extent of any change in bowel movement frequency should be obtained. It has been demonstrated in a palliative care population that the objective assessment of stool appearance correlates well with bowel transit time.[27] This is a noninvasive, technology-free method of assessing a key indicator of intestinal function, but nonetheless it is likely to be used by clinicians only in support of a particular audit or research inquiry.

A simple objective indicator of the presence of constipation is a plain abdominal radiograph. A scoring system to describe the amount of stool present was described and tested by Bruera et al. in palliative care patients.[28] Similar systems of more or less complexity have been described by Barr[29] and others in different populations, and claim to show high interobserver reliability and good correlation with stool frequency.

Radiographs are a static measure of current fecal loading and give no information about the speed of transit or about performance of different colonic segments. Scoring of pre- and postintervention radiographs could at least aid objectivity in the assessment of the effectiveness of interventions to clear a constipated bowel. On the other hand, there is no indication for making an abdominal radiograph a routine part of patient assessment. In practice, its principal role is to help distinguish between constipation and intestinal obstruction in cases where doubt exists on the basis of clinical assessment.

Blood tests do not, of course, indicate anything about the presence or severity of constipation, but hypercalcemia of malignancy can be a contributory factor in the condition and should be tested for.

Subjective Assessments

Subjective measures of constipation, which assess patients' reports of their bowel function without externally measurable criteria, take the form of visual analog (VAS) or adjectival scales, or of questionnaires. A discrete response modification of the VAS and an adjectival scale have each been found to have validity and are easy to use in a palliative care setting.[30] Since the main cause of diarrhea in palliative care is excessive use of laxatives to treat constipation, it is appropriate that any subjective measure includes the ability to assess not only constipation but also diarrhea as well. This is easily arranged with VAS and adjectival scales, but it is lacking in the questionnaires that have been validated for the assessment of constipation.

Perhaps the best established constipation questionnaire is the Constipation Assessment Scale (CAS) of McMillan and Williams.[31] This is an eight-item scale validated on cancer patients. Completion time averages two minutes.

The Patient Assessment of Constipation Symptom Questionnaire (PAC-SYM) and the Patient Assessment of Constipation Quality of Life Questionnaire (PAC-QOL) are related questionnaires directed at the patient's perspective on constipation.[32] The PAC-SYM has three subscales related to stool symptoms, rectal symptoms, and abdominal symptoms respectively, and has been validated on a large ($n = 216$) sample of chronically constipated subjects but not a cancer population. The PAC-QOL is a constipation-specific quality-of-life measure. The PAC-SYM contains no assessment of diarrhea, although the PAC-QOL has a bowel frequency rating. Several other bowel function rating scales exist, but they are either derived from one of those already mentioned or are not specific to constipation.

Examination

Abdominal examination and, unless there has been a recent full evacuation, rectal examination are vital, and will help to avoid the following major errors in the diagnosis of constipation:

- *Impaction, presenting as diarrhea, often with incontinence.* This occurs characteristically in elderly patients in whom inattention to the need to defecate, confusion, or rectal insensitivity leads to the formation of a large fecal mass, which is impossible to pass spontaneously. Fecal material higher in the colon is broken down into semiliquid form by bacterial action and seeps past the mass, appearing as diarrhea and, if the closing pressure of the anal sphincters has been exceeded by the mass, fecal leakage or incontinence. Nearly all fecal impactions are said to occur in the rectum and can be diagnosed on rectal examination.

- *Intestinal obstruction by tumor or adhesions.* Known intra-abdominal malignant deposits, previous intestinal surgery, alternating constipation and diarrhea, gut colic, and nausea and vomiting combine to suggest the presence of intestinal obstruction. A similar picture can, however, occur in severe constipation. The distinction is important, in case of obstruction, as attempts to clear "constipation" by use of stimulant laxatives can cause severe pain.
- *Nausea.* Some patients rapidly experience nausea, with or without vomiting, in the presence of intestinal holdup. Unexplained nausea or vomiting should prompt inquiry and examination for constipation.
- *Abdominal pain.* The effort of colonic muscle to propel hard feces commonly leads to abdominal pain, frequently colicky in nature. History and examination usually suggest the cause of the pain, but constipation is still sometimes "treated" with morphine. Such pain may be particularly marked—and difficult to diagnose—where abdominal or pelvic tumor exists, presumably as a result either of pressure on the tumor from distended gut or because of partial intestinal obstruction.
- *Urinary incontinence.* Fecal impaction is well recognized as a precipitant of urinary incontinence in the elderly, and the recent onset of incontinence should indicate abdominal and rectal examination as the first investigative steps.

Palpation of the abdomen may reveal fecal masses in the line of the descending colon and even that of the more proximal colon and cecum. The distinction between tumor and fecal masses can be hard to make. Feces will usually indent, if the patient will tolerate sufficiently firm pressure, and may give a crepitus-like sensation because of entrained gas. Sometimes an abdominal radiograph is needed to distinguish tumor from stool, but this is uncommon. Digital examination of the rectum may reveal a hard mass of impacted feces. The clinical picture, however, may be of fecal leakage. Alternatively, the complete absence of stool implies colonic inertia.

Rectal examination may also uncover rectal tumor, a rectocele, solitary rectal ulcer, or anal stenosis. A lax anal sphincter may indicate spinal cord damage associated with colonic hypotonia. If a rectocele or compression from pelvic tumor masses is suspected, vaginal examination may be justifiable. Examination of the stool can be useful. Small, hard pellets suggest slow colonic transit; ribbonlike stools suggest stenosis or hemorrhoids; and blood or mucus suggest tumor, hemorrhoids, or coexisting colitis.

MANAGEMENT

Prophylaxis

It is much better to prevent constipation than to treat it only after it has occurred. The etiologies of constipation in patients with cancer (see Table 5.1) suggest several prophylactic measures. First, good general symptom control should exist, without which no other measures are possible. A key stimulus to colonic peristalsis and defecation is activity.[33] Hence, patients should be encouraged and enabled to be as mobile as their physical limitations allow.

Constipated stools have relatively low water content, rendering them hard and difficult to pass. This tendency will be exacerbated if the individual is dehydrated, and an adequate fluid intake is therefore helpful.

Ill people have small appetites and what food they do eat tends to be low in fiber. Dietary fiber deficiency has been linked with constipation in Western society, but individuals with severe constipation are not fiber deficient and their gut function responds poorly to added fiber.[34] Work with radiotherapy patients in Oxford suggested that an increase in stool frequency of 50 percent would require an approximately 450 percent mean increase in dietary fiber, well beyond the tolerance of most subjects.[35] Hence, although opportunities should be taken to raise the fiber content of patients' diets, this alone will not correct severe constipation and the priority remains that food should be as attractive as possible to the person who is expected to eat it.

There should be awareness of which drugs are likely to cause constipation. Apart from opioids, key culprits in palliative care are anticholinergics and drugs that show some anticholinergic effects, such as psychotropics, antidepressants, and some antiemetics. The most effective approach is avoidance, but this is often not practicable, in which case a laxative should be prescribed from the outset, without waiting until constipation is established.

Institutional lack of privacy for defecation and the use of bedpans, which impose an inappropriate posture and greatly increase the pressure required to expel a stool, create an environment conducive to constipation. Evidence suggests that practiced patients adapt to such indignities, but it should be a priority to allow patients privacy and the use of a bathroom, or at least a commode, for defecation.

Complementary Therapies

Many patients express interest in complementary approaches to the management of constipation, including herbal remedies, reflexology, and abdominal massage. Several herbal preparations, such as rhubarb, chrysanthemum stems, and peach leaves, are known to contain substances with properties similar to stimulant laxatives marketed by the pharmaceutical industry.

There are also preparations of regional interest. An ayurvedic medicine has been demonstrated in an Indian study to have efficacy rivaling that of senna.[36] From Argentina there is uncontrolled evidence for the laxative effectiveness of baker's yeast for constipation in palliative care.[37]

A small within-subject trial of sham versus true acupuncture in chronically constipated children found an increase in stool frequency during the true acupuncture phase.[38] However, despite the popularity of acupuncture for management of pain and, to a lesser extent, nausea in palliative care, there appear to have been no trials of its use for constipation in terminally ill adults.

Abdominal massage is a time-honored management of constipation in which there has been increasing recent interest. A trial of abdominal massage in constipated adults did as well as the prevailing not very effective laxative regime, but consumed considerable resources in staff time.[39] Other trials of the technique have been small, poorly designed, and inconclusive.[40] In general, however, there is a lack of evidence regarding the effectiveness of complementary techniques for the management of bowel dysfunction or other symptoms in palliative care.

Laxative Therapy

The basic division of laxatives is between stimulants and softeners (see Figure 5.1). This division seems useful in clinical practice, al-

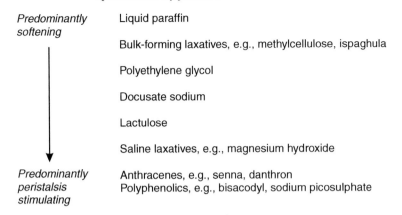

Predominantly softening

Liquid paraffin

Bulk-forming laxatives, e.g., methylcellulose, ispaghula

Polyethylene glycol

Docusate sodium

Lactulose

Saline laxatives, e.g., magnesium hydroxide

Predominantly peristalsis stimulating

Anthracenes, e.g., senna, danthron
Polyphenolics, e.g., bisacodyl, sodium picosulphate

FIGURE 5.1. Oral laxative classification. *Source:* Adapted from Sykes NP. Constipation and Diarrhoea. In Doyle D, Hanks G, Cherney N, and Kenneth C (eds.), *Oxford textbook of palliative medicine,* Third edition. Oxford: Oxford University Press, 2003:513-526. By permission of Oxford University Press.

though in fact any drug that stimulates peristalsis will accelerate transit, allow less time for water absorption, and so produce a softer stool. Similarly, softening the stool involves increasing its bulk, which will result in increased distension of the intestinal wall and a consequent stimulation of reflex enteric muscle contraction.

Most trials of laxative drugs have been carried out in gastroenterology or in geriatrics. The results do not allow a clear recommendation of one agent over another because of the small size of the studies, the number of different preparations, and the various end points and conditions involved. Indeed, it has been suggested that the quality of the evidence even in chronic constipation is too poor to allow conclusions to be drawn about the efficacy of laxatives.[41]

However, if a less nihilistic view is taken, certain statements can be made:

• Systematic review evidence suggests that any kind of laxative can increase stool frequency by about 1.4 bowel actions per week compared with placebo.[42]
• A volunteer trial used either a softening laxative, a stimulant laxative, or a combination preparation to counteract the constipation caused by loperamide as a source of opioid-induced con-

stipation. It concluded that the optimal combination of effectiveness with minimum adverse effects and medication burden was achieved by using a combination of stimulant and softening laxatives rather than either alone.[43]

• Laxative preparations vary significantly in price and physical characteristics. Ready-made combinations tend to be expensive. In the United States spending on laxatives exceeds $500 million annually. Given the lack of major differences in efficacy, cost and individual patient acceptability should both be strong influences in prescribing choice.[44]

The aim of laxative therapy is comfortable defecation, not any particular frequency of evacuation. No single laxative dose is adequate for everyone, and many patients are subjected to both rectal interventions and an inadequate oral dose of laxative. The dose needs to be titrated against the response and the advent of adverse effects, remembering the latent period of action of the drug concerned, and should be increased prophylactically if, say, opioids are introduced or their dose is being substantially increased.

Oral Laxatives

Stimulant laxatives. Examples include senna, bisacodyl, sodium picosulfate, danthron (only available in combination preparations). Common starting doses are senna 15 mg daily; bisacodyl 10 mg daily; sodium picosulphate 5 mg daily; and danthron 50 mg daily. These laxatives

• act directly on the myenteric nerves to evoke gut muscle contraction;
• reduce gut water absorption;
• can produce marked colic, particularly if not combined with a softening agent; and
• have an onset of action of 6 to 12 hours.

Danthron causes red urinary discoloration and perianal rashes. Animal testing using large doses has suggested the possibility of carcinogenicity, and for this reason danthron-containing products are licensed in the United Kingdom only for use in palliative care. In fact, similar suspicions exist about the stimulant laxatives as a group, because of an association between their chronic use and the appearance of a dark staining of the gut mucosa, termed *melanosis coli,* that has been proposed to be a premalignant condition. However, a large (n = 440) prospective study found no association between anthranoid laxative use or melanosis coli and either adenoma or carcinoma of the colon.[45] Similarly, a lack of association has been found between anthranoid laxative intake, melanosis coli and the presence of aberrant crypt foci, which are areas of intestinal mucosa showing premalignant change.[46] It therefore appears likely that the cancer-inducing dangers of these agents have been overstated. Chronic usage is also said to be associated with neuronal loss in the myenteric plexus, a process that is postulated to be responsible for tolerance to the laxatives. Again, experimental studies have failed to confirm that exposure to these drugs actually produces such damage.[47]

Softening laxatives. These can be divided into four groups: osmotic, surfactant, and lubricant laxatives, as well as bulking agents.

1. *Osmotic laxatives* include magnesium sulfate, magnesium hydroxide, lactulose, and polyethylene glycol (PEG). Common starting doses are magnesium hydroxide or sulfate 2 to 4 g daily; lactulose 15 mL b.i.d.; polyethylene glycol 1 sachet in 125 mL water daily (fecal impaction 8 sachets in 1 liter of water over 6 hours).

Magnesium sulfate and hydroxide have stimulant as well as osmotic actions at higher doses. The sulfate is the more potent. They are inexpensive. Magnesium sulfate used alone can be useful for resistant constipation. There is a risk of hypermagnesemia with chronic use. Magnesium hydroxide is less potent than the sulfate and, either alone or as an emulsion with liquid paraffin, deserves reevaluation as a less expensive alternative to lactulose and other more popular preparations.[48]

Lactulose is not broken down or absorbed in the small gut, where, as a result, it exerts an osmotic influence to retain water in the lumen. Bacterial degradation in the colon produces short-chain organic acids that lower the intestinal pH, possibly stimulating peristalsis, and increasing stool bulk by enlargement of the microbial mass. These acids are absorbed and so the osmotic effect does not extend throughout the colon. Mannitol and sorbitol work similarly, the latter having been reported to be as effective as lactulose, less costly, and less likely to be nauseating.[49] Some drawbacks are listed here:

- It is expensive. In the United Kingdom, a single hospital saved the equivalent of $45,000 over two years by removing lactulose from its formulary.
- It is needed in large volumes if used alone in marked constipation.
- It causes flatulence in around 20 percent of users.

PEG is a nonabsorbed, nondegraded polymer prepared in solution (which may be rendered isoosmotic with sodium bicarbonate and sodium and potassium chlorides to avoid electrolyte disturbance). It provides a source of nonabsorbed fluid that can then exert a softening effect on the bowel contents. Stool weight is increased in proportion to the total mass of PEG ingested and gut transit is accelerated. PEG has been reported to be effective as an oral treatment for fecal impaction[50] or, indeed, as a single dose treatment for chronic constipation.[51] However, it then has to be taken in substantial volumes (500 to 1,000 mL per day), which can prove unacceptable to more frail patients. The raised osmotic pressure in the gut produced by PEG has been found to inhibit proliferation of colonic cancer cells in animal models.[52] Whether this observation has clinical relevance remains to be determined.

2. *Surfactant laxatives* include docusate sodium and poloxamer (available in United Kingdom only in combination with dantron). The common starting dose is docusate sodium 300 mg daily.

These drugs act as detergents to increase water penetration, and hence softening, of the stool. Docusate also promotes water, sodium, and chloride secretion in the jejunum and colon. There is a clinical impression that at higher doses it may stimulate peristalsis. Evidence for laxative efficacy is limited.

3. A *lubricant laxative* is liquid paraffin, with a typical starting dose of 10 mL daily.

The possibility of liquid paraffin causing fat-soluble vitamin deficiencies has probably been exaggerated and is not relevant to palliative care. However, its use has been associated with troublesome anal fecal leakage. No adverse effects have been linked with the emulsion of 25 percent liquid paraffin with 75 percent magnesium hydroxide, which is currently the most common form in which it is used in Britain. It is a less expensive choice.

4. *Bulking agents* include bran, methylcellulose, and ispaghula. Typical starting doses are bran 8 g daily, others 3 to 4 g daily.

Bulking agents are "normalizers" rather than true laxatives: they will soften a hard stool but make firmer a loose one. Stool bulk is increased partly by providing material that resists bacterial breakdown and hence remains in the gut, and partly by providing a substrate for bacterial growth and gas production. It appears that transit is speeded especially as a result of fermentation and is to some degree independent of stool bulking action.[53]

Effective in mild constipation, but probably not in severe constipation, they need to be taken with ample water (at least 200 to 300 mL); this and their consistency are unacceptable to many ill patients. If taken with inadequate water, a viscous mass may result which can precipitate intestinal tract obstruction. Use of bulking agents is therefore inappropriate in patients whose disease puts them at risk of bowel obstruction.

Rectal Laxatives

Most patients prefer oral laxatives to rectal. Hence, the use of suppositories and enemas should be minimized by optimizing laxative treatment by mouth. There is, however, a particular role for enemas and suppositories in the relief of fecal impaction and in bowel management in patients whose neurological dysfunction is resulting in fecal incontinence. Evidence to guide their use is scantier even than that for oral laxatives. Anything introduced into the rectum can stimulate defecation via the anocolonic reflex, but among rectal laxatives only bisacodyl suppositories have a pharmacological stimulant action. Glycerine suppositories, and arachis or olive oil enemas, soften and lubricate the stool, as do proprietary minienemas, which contain mixtures of surfactants.

An Approach to the Management of Constipation

There are insufficient data on the management of constipation for proper evidence-based guidelines to be produced. However, the following approach is in accord with such evidence as does exist:

- Rectal examination is needed unless there has been a recent complete bowel action.

- If the rectum is impacted with hard feces, it might be necessary to soften the mass with an oil retention enema before evacuation is possible.
- If manual rectal evacuation proves necessary, ensure adequate sedation with diazepam or midazolam.
- If the rectum is loaded with soft feces, an oral stimulant laxative alone may be adequate. The addition of a softener is likely to be needed in due course.
- If the rectum is largely empty, a combination of softening and stimulant laxatives should be given and the doses titrated according to response. Particularly when opioids are also being given, a b.i.d. or t.i.d. laxative dose schedule is likely to be needed. Remember patient acceptability and cost.
- The bowel frequency to be aimed at is one that the individual patient is happy with, but clinically it seems that an interval of more than three days between bowel actions is more likely to be associated with subsequent difficulty in defecation.
- There is no clear hierarchy of laxatives, but sodium picosulfate or magnesium sulfate appear helpful for more resistant constipation.
- In general, (1) seek to maximize activity; (2) encourage an adequate fluid intake; and (3) encourage as high a fiber content to the diet as the person can comfortably manage.

New Laxative Developments

There is much scope for further work on the comparative efficacy and palatability of conventional laxatives. However, several new developments are worth mentioning.

There is interest in the use of prokinetic agents to accelerate intestinal transit. Cisapride, which acts by enhancing acetylcholine release from myenteric neurones through $5HT_4$ receptor agonism, is better than placebo in improving stool consistency and frequency in idiopathic constipation,[54] but has been associated with significant cardiotoxicity. The more recent prucalopride has similar effects and enhances rectal sensitivity, a property that may be of particular relevance to patients taking opioids.[55] Tegaserod is another recent $5HT_4$ agonist that has been found to improve constipation, this time in irritable bowel syndrome.[56] It is perhaps doubtful whether this class of agent will be effective alone against opioid-induced constipation, but they may be able to act as "colaxatives" to enhance the effect of conventional laxatives given alongside. Metoclopramide, which also increases gastrointestinal motility by interaction with gut $5HT_4$ receptors, has been shown to be effective in narcotic bowel syndrome when given by continuous subcutaneous infusion[1]. Oral metoclopramide has not found a place in routine laxative treatment, and it is less potently prokinetic than cisapride.

As an antibiotic, oral erythromycin causes diarrhea on about 50 percent of occasions. Apart from altering the balance of the gut flora, erythromycin acts as an agonist at motilin receptors, which are responsible for initiating the migrating motor complex in the small bowel. Motilin receptors are also present elsewhere in the gut, and erythromycin reduces transit time in the right colon in healthy humans.[57] However, colonic activity was not stimulated in a group of chronically constipated individuals,[58] and so whether erythromycin and related macrolides that also possess a 14-carbon lactone ring will be effective laxatives or predominantly antireflux agents remains to be seen.

Probiotics have been proposed as potentially valuable in both constipation and diarrhea through modification of gut flora and, indirectly, of motility. In a small ($n = 28$) controlled trial in elderly patients, the addition of *Lactobacillus rhamnosus* and *Propionibacterium freudenreichii* to the diet showed a modest increase in stool frequency but no reduction in laxative use.[59]

Morphine-induced constipation can be counteracted by an opioid antagonist given orally because a major part of the opioid effect on the human gut is mediated peripherally rather than centrally. This subject is dealt with fully in other chapters.

NAUSEA AND VOMITING

Nausea affects up to 70 percent of patients with advanced cancer and vomiting affects 10 to 30 percent.[60] Table 5.2 indicates that the potential causes are many and are certainly not limited to opioids even in those who take them. Nonetheless, morphine has been said to cause nausea and vomiting in as many as 70 percent of patients as

TABLE 5.2. Common causes of nausea and vomiting in advanced cancer.

Category	Cause
Gastrointestinal	Gastritis (aocohol, NSAIDs)
	Gastric outlet obstruction (tumor, fibrosis, functional)
	Slow gastric emptying (autonomic gastropathy, functional, drugs)
	Squashed stomach syndrome (hepatomegaly, ascites, linitis plastica)
	Intestinal obstruction
	Constipation
Drugs	Opioids
	Digoxin
	Theophyllines
	Cytotoxics
	Erythromycin
Metabolic	Renal failure
	Hypercalcemia
	Hyponatremia
Neurological	Raised intracranial pressure
	Posterior fossa tumors
	Meningeal infiltration
	Skull metastases
Emotional	Anxiety
	Anticipatory vomiting with chemotherapy
Other	Severe uncontrolled pain
	Colic of any origin
	Radiotherapy: especially to L1 region, high dose brain radiotherapy, upper hemibody radiation
	Cough, thick sputum, postnasal drip

Source: Adapted from Sykes N, Pace V. Control of symptoms other than pain. In Sykes N, Fallon MT, Patt RB (eds.), *Clinical pain management: Cancer pain.* London: Arnold, 2003:293-318. Copyright © 2003 by Arnold. Reproduced by permission of Edward Arnold.

they start the drug.[60] However, clinical experience indicates that tolerance to this adverse effect occurs rapidly and the problem resolves over three or four days. It also appears that in both animals and man, lower morphine doses are more emetogenic than higher ones.[61]

The Mechanisms of Opioids' Emetic Action

Morphine, and by implication other μ-acting opioids, acts in at least three ways to cause nausea and vomiting:

1. Detection by the chemoreceptor trigger area in the region of the area postrema and nucleus tractus solitarius, both situated in the hindbrain close to the fourth ventricle
2. Slowing of gastrointestinal transit and, in particular, gastric emptying (In contrast to the pyloric sphincter spasm seen in animals, the mechanism of gastric emptying delay in man appears to be contraction of the proximal duodenum.[62] The resulting gastric distension causes emetogenic inputs via 5HT release in the gut and transmission centrally via the vagus.)
3. Increase of vestibular sensitivity (The principal evidence for this is the observation that ambulatory patients are more likely to vomit than bedfast ones.)

Vomiting consists of a complex series of coordinated events. Autonomic changes, retching, and hypersalivation occur. These are followed by simultaneous contraction of abdominal and diaphragmatic muscles and relaxation of sphincters, together with closure of the epiglottis and nasopharynx as the vomit is expelled. These actions are choreographed by the integrative vomiting center, sometimes known as the emetic pattern generator, in order to emphasize the fact that rather than being a discrete structure, it consists of a number of medullary nuclei. These have separate functions but, when occasion requires, act in concert to orchestrate the act of vomiting.

The various nuclei involved in vomiting differ in their predominant populations of neurotransmitters (see Figure 5.2), although each nucleus is mixed and a considerable number of receptor types are known to be represented. Antiemetic drugs are neurotransmitter blocking agents, and this raises the possibility that if the nuclei predominantly involved in mediating a particular instance of vomiting can be identified, a drug can be chosen that blocks the principal neurotransmitters in those areas. In this way the chance of achieving emetic control will be maximized. This theory underlies the rational approach to antiemesis practiced in palliative care. Unfortunately, in

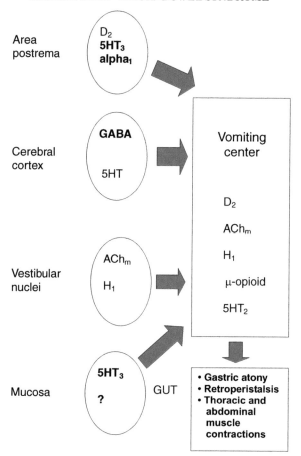

FIGURE 5.2. Schematic representation of the neurophysiology of vomiting.

real life it is often difficult to identify a single cause of nausea and vomiting and probably in most cases there are multiple causes.

Management of Opioid-Induced Nausea and Vomiting

A first step is to ensure that the patient is actually vomiting rather than regurgitating, as the latter will not be helped by antiemetics. The presence of neurological or malignant disease affecting the esophagus should raise suspicions that regurgitation may be occurring. Undigested food of the kind being eaten in a current or immediately past meal returned in small volumes with little or no prodromal nausea suggests regurgitation.

Several measures of nausea and vomiting are available but there is no agreed standard, making comparison of study results difficult.[60] A preliminary in any confirmed case of nausea or vomiting is to consider and address the existence of exacerbating factors such as strong smells, anxiety, and, of course, constipation. At least 30 percent of patients receiving morphine do not need an antiemetic, but around 10 percent will need a combination of two or more antiemetics.[63] The logical choice of antiemetic depends on which of the three mechanisms of opioid-induced emesis appears to be acting most strongly. In practice, vestibular stimulation can be ignored unless the patient has to take a journey, as movement per se is not usually the sole stimulus to nausea and vomiting in this patient group. Table 5.3 shows the sites and relative potencies of receptor action of commonly used antiemetics.

Delayed gastric emptying is suggested by large volume vomits, containing little or no bile, occurring suddenly with little or no preceding nausea. There may be complaints of hiccups and heartburn,

TABLE 5.3. Receptor activity of commonly used antiemetics.

Antiemetic	D_2	ACh_m	H_1	$5HT_3$	$5HT_4$
Hyoscine	–	+++	–	–	–
Cyclizine	–	+	+++	–	–
Haloperidol	+++	–	–	–	–
Chlorpromazine	++	+	++	–	–
Metoclopramide	++	–	–	+	++
Domperidone	++	–	–	–	–
Ondansetron	–	–	–	+++	+
Levomepromazine	++	+	+	+	–
Droperidol	+++	–	–	–	–

–: Indicates little or no activity.
+++: Indicates strong antagonism.

and there is often undigested food in the vomit from meals taken more than six hours previously. In this situation metoclopramide is the rational first choice of antiemetic because of its prokinetic action on the upper gut. Metoclopramide has been shown to overcome opioid-related upper gut slowing and associated vomiting.[64] Other prokinetics, such as the now-withdrawn cisapride and the more recent prucalopride and tegaserod, have been shown to enhance gastric emptying perhaps more potently than metoclopramide, but their effect seems stronger on symptoms of reflux than on nausea and vomiting. Uniquely, metoclopramide has not only the $5HT_4$ agonist activity that endows it with its prokinetic properties but also central antidopaminergic activity at D_2 receptors and, at high doses, $5HT_3$ antagonism. This combination of properties theoretically allows the drug to intercept the emetogenic action of opioids both peripherally and centrally. However, since its central antidopaminergic action is less potent than that of some other agents, in particular haloperidol, it is the first choice only when peripheral mechanisms of vomiting are apparent. A controlled release version of metoclopramide has been shown to be more effective in cancer-related nausea with dyspepsia than an immediate release formulation.[65] As with any antiemetic in a vomiting patient, efficacy is likely to be better if metoclopramide is administered by continuous subcutaneous infusion. The usual dose ranges in palliative care are 10 to 20 mg t.i.d. IR, 15 to 30 mg b.i.d. MR, or 30 to 120 mg per 24 hours subcutaneously. Higher doses have been used to accompany cytotoxic chemotherapy regimes.

Domperidone, not available in the United States, is a peripheral dopamine antagonist that is sometimes regarded clinically as an alternative to metoclopramide. It influences upper gut dopaminergic tone to enhance the coordination of antral-duodenal motility. In practice domperidone is perhaps best regarded as an antidopaminergic agent whose lack of central effects should render it less likely to precipitate or exacerbate dystonic or Parkinsonian symptoms in vulnerable patients. These are adverse effects that metoclopramide can certainly cause, especially if combined with another antidopaminergic drug.

The chemoreceptor areas involved in emetogenesis are rich in D_2 dopamine receptors and, in the absence of evidence of gastric holdup, it is appropriate to use a drug with antidopaminergic activity for opioid-related nausea or vomiting. The most potent and specific antidopaminergics are droperidol and haloperidol. Droperidol is short acting, but haloperidol has a half-life of about 18 hours, rendering it suitable initially to be given once a day, usually in the evening (1.5 mg nocte) because of its relatively mild sedative effects. A systematic review of the use of haloperidol as an antiemetic in palliative care found evidence of effectiveness in nausea and vomiting of a variety of causes, including morphine. As often in the field, though, the studies were few and of mediocre quality.[66] The dose of haloperidol can be titrated upward to a total of 10 mg per day, and it can be administered by subcutaneous infusion. However, by this dose level the sedative and sometimes the extrapyramidal or Parkinsonian effects of haloperidol tend to appear and a change of drug or combination with a complementary antiemetic is appropriate.

In British palliative care a popular antiemetic to use at this point to replace haloperidol is levomepromazine (methotrimeprazine), because of its broad spectrum of action which can cover the mixed etiology of vomiting so often found in this patient group. Levomepromazine is a phenothiazine with pronounced sedative and some analgesic effects. A major evolution in its use has been the demonstration that its antiemetic effectiveness extends to much lower doses than previously assumed, allowing it to be used without creating troublesome drowsiness.[67] Current usual doses are 6.25 to 25 mg per day orally or 2.5 to 12.5 mg per day subcutaneously. The risk of extrapyramidal effects is lower than with haloperidol, but is not absent.

In view of the spectrum of their receptor activities it is possible that the newer atypical antipsychotic drugs, which have a more benign adverse effect profile than older neuroleptics, might be effective antiemetics against opioid-induced vomiting. A preliminary trial using olanzapine, whose receptor profile resembles that of levomepromazine, in cancer patients receiving opioid analgesia showed significant antiemetic benefits over placebo with no evidence of extrapyramidal or Parkinsonian effects and no mental slowing.[68] Larger, blinded studies are awaited of this drug and of risperidone, whose activity profile is somewhat different.

Cyclizine is an older, cheap drug that offers a range of receptor activities complementary to those of haloperidol and has been used for many years to control emesis associated with analgesics.[69] In nausea and vomiting associated with patient-controlled opioid analgesia postoperatively, cyclizine has been found to have efficacy comparable with that of droperidol.[70] Its H_1 antihistaminic activity suggests a role at vagal level, which would be relevant where nausea was associated with gut distension. Cyclizine has tended to be used both as a general purpose antiemetic in palliative care and, more specifically, in vomiting associated with bowel obstruction. A standard dose of 50 mg t.i.d. or 150 mg per 24 hours subcutaneously is used. In theory cyclizine's anticholinergic actions would tend to antagonize the prokinetic effects of metoclopramide where these were important. Research evidence of the clinical importance of this effect is lacking.

The advent of specific $5HT_3$ receptor antagonists has had a major impact on antiemesis for cancer chemotherapy. Some 80 percent of the body's serotonin is contained in the gut wall, and elevated levels of circulating serotonin are associated with gut distension due to malignant intestinal obstruction. $5HT_3$ receptors are present in the vagus, which provides central inputs from the upper gut and in the area postrema. It is therefore plausible that $5HT_3$ antagonists might have a role in combating opioid-related vomiting via either chemoreceptor or gastric slowing mechanisms. A case report from a palliative care setting indicated that for a patient with a complex vomiting etiology, the combination of ondansetron and haloperidol was better than either alone.[71] Other similar case history reports on palliative cancer patients exist, but randomized, controlled trials in the prevention of opioid-related vomiting in the postoperative situation have produced mixed results. Hence, the place of $5HT_3$ antagonists in morphine-induced vomiting remains unclear. The high cost of these drugs, however, is perfectly apparent.

Steroids have no specific effect against opioid-related nausea and vomiting, and have cumulative and serious adverse effects. Cannabinoids tend to produce marked sedation when used in combination with opioids in ill patients. In consequence, neither of these drug groups has found wide favor as antiemetics in palliative care.

Alternative Antiemetics

Among physicians is much interest in developing new types of antiemetic drugs. Closest to the market are the NK_1 receptor antagonists, but clinical trials to date indicate a lack of activity of these drugs in opioid-induced vomiting.[72]

Among patients there is interest in nondrug approaches to antiemesis, notably acupuncture and acupressure. Controlled trial evidence from surgical patients suggests that acupuncture at the P6 point (just above the wrist) is more effective than placebo for the control of nausea and vomiting due to opioid premedication.[73] This finding has been replicated widely in the same setting for conventional acupuncture, electroacupuncture (including transcutaneous electrical nerve stimulation), and acupressure using proprietary wrist bands to exert pressure over the P6 point. A meta-analysis concluded that in postoperative nausea and vomiting these techniques offered efficacy comparable to commonly used antiemetics.[74] No studies have specifically tested these therapies against opioid-related nausea and vomiting in a palliative care context.

Reducing the Emetic Effects of Opioids

There is potential for reducing the degree of nausea and vomiting experienced from opioid analgesia either by changing the opioid used or the route by which it is administered. In relation to the route of morphine administration, studies are small but tend to show lower rates of emesis with nonoral routes compared to giving the drug by mouth.[60] Similar evidence is not available for other opioids.

Oxycodone,[23] hydromorphone,[24] and methadone[75] have been reported to be less emetogenic than morphine, but no difference was found between the frequencies of nausea caused by fentanyl and subcutaneous morphine.[76] It has to be recognized that the size of most of the studies is small. On the basis of trials totaling over 16,000 subjects, tramadol has been found to have an incidence of nausea and vomiting of just over 4 percent, considerably lower than reported levels for morphine.[25] However, the analgesic abilities of these two drugs are not equivalent and it would frequently be impracticable to change a patient from morphine to tramadol.

Switching from one opioid to another has been reported to improve analgesia and a range of adverse effects, including nausea but also, particularly, confusion. It is increasingly clear that as well as intrinsic differences between opioid drugs in terms of their affinities for subtypes of opioid receptors and their active metabolites, individuals' genetic constitutions produce significant variation in the patterns of opioid receptor subtypes that the body exhibits. In consequence it is easy to envisage that responses to opioids will be idiosyncratic and, at this stage of our knowledge, impossible to forecast. If a patient tolerates an opioid poorly, a change to any other opioid of equivalent potency may produce better analgesia and fewer side effects, including nausea.

CONCLUSION

In palliative care opioid bowel dysfunction is an important contributor to nausea and vomiting and to constipation, but both groups of symptoms are generally multifactorial. This renders defining a specific treatment difficult. However, both sets of symptoms cause great distress to many patients, and it is vital for clinicians to be capable of assessing each symptom adequately and to be aware of the therapeutic options available. More research would always be welcome, but much could be achieved now by better patient information, attention to detail on the part of attending physicians and nurses, and persistance in efforts to achieve the highest degree of relief possible against a clinical background that is ever changing and usually deteriorating.

NOTES

1. Bruera E, Brenneis C, Michand M, MacDonald N. Continuous subcutaneous infusion of metoclopramide for treatment of narcotic bowel syndrome. *Cancer Treat Rep* 1987;71:1121-1122.

2. Donaldson AN. Experimental study of intestinal stasis. *JAMA* 1922;78: 884-888.

3. Ventafridda V, Oliveri E, Caraceni A, Spoldi E, de Conno F, Saita L, Ripamonti C. A retrospective study on the use of oral morphine in cancer pain. *J Pain Symptom Manage* 1987;2:77-81.

4. Dunlop GM. A study of the relative frequency and importance of gastrointestinal symptoms and weakness in patients with far advanced cancer: Student paper. *Palliat Med* 1989;4:37-44.

5. Holmes S. Use of a modified symptom distress scale in assessment of the cancer patient. *Int J Nurs Stud* 1989;26:69-79.

6. Thompson WG, Longstreth GF, Drossman DA, Heaton KW, Irvine EJ, Müller-Lissner SA. Functional bowel disorders and functional abdominal pain. *Gut* 1999;45:1143-1147.

7. Drossman D A, Sandler R S, McKee D C, Lovitz A J. Bowel patterns among subjects not seeking health care. *Gastroenterology* 1982;83:529-534.

8. Connell A M, Hilton C, Irvine G, Lennard-Jones J E, Misiewicz J J. Variation in bowel habit in two population samples. *Brit Med J* 1965;ii:1095-1099.

9. Herz MJ, Kahan E, Zalevski S, Aframian R, Kuznitz D, Reichman S. Constipation: a different entity for patients and doctors. *Fam Pract* 1996;13:156-159.

10. Ashraf W, Park F, Lof J, Quigley EM. An examination of the reliability of reported stool frequency in the diagnosis of idiopathic constipation. *Amer J Gastroenterol* 1996;91:26-32.

11. Thompson WG, Heaton KW. Functional bowel disorders in apparently healthy people. *Gastroenterology* 1980;79:283-288.

12. Everhart J E, Go V L, Johannes R S, Fitzsimmons S C, Roth H P, White L R. A longitudinal survey of self-reported bowel habits in the United States. *Digest Dis Sci* 1989;34:1153-1162.

13. Wigzell F W. The health of nonagenarians. *Gerontol Clin (Basel)* 1969;11: 137-144.

14. Cartwright A, Hockey L, Anderson JL. *Life before death.* London: Routledge and Kegan Paul; 1973:23.

15. Smith S. Evidence-based management of constipation in the oncology patient. *Eur J Oncol Nurs* 2001;5:18-25.

16. Johanson JF, Sonnenberrg A, Koch TR, McCarty DJ. Association of constipation with neurologic diseases. *Digest Dis Sci* 1992;37:179-186.

17. Hennessey A, Robertson NP, Swingler R, Compston DA. Urinary, faecal and sexual dysfunction in patients with multiple sclerosis. *J Neurol* 1999;246:1027-1032.

18. Robinson CB, Fritch M, Hullett L, Petersen MA, Sikkema S, Theuninck L, Timmer K. Development of a protocol to prevent opioid-induced constipation in patients with cancer: A research utilization project. *Clin J Oncol Nurs* 2000;4(2): 79-84.

19. Sykes NP. The relationship between opioid use and laxative use in terminally ill cancer patients. *Palliat Med* 1998;12:375-382.

20. Ling GS, Paul D, Simontov R, Pasternak GW. Differential development of acute tolerance. *Life Sci* 1989;45:1627-1636.

21. Fallon M, Hanks G. Morphine, constipation and performance status in advanced cancer patients. *Palliat Med* 1999;13:159-160.

22. Radbruch L, Sabatowski R, Loick G, Kulbe C, Kasper M, Grond S, Lehmann KA. Constipation and the use of laxatives: A comparison between transdermal fentanyl and oral morphine. *Palliat Med* 2000;14:111-119.

23. Daeninck PJ, Bruera E. Reduction in constipation and laxative requirements following opioid rotation to methadone. *J Pain Symptom Manage* 1999;18:303-309.

24. Poyhia R, Vainio A, Kalso E. A review of oxycodone's pharmacokinetics and pharmacodynamics. *J Pain Symptom Manage* 1993;8:63-67.

25. Sarhill N, Walsh D, Nelson KA. Hydromorphone: Pharmacology and clinical applications in cancer patients. *Support Care Cancer* 2001;9:84-96.

26. Lee CR, McTavish D, Sorkin EM. Tramadol: A preliminary review of its pharmacodynamic and pharmacokinetic properties, and therapeutic potential in various acute and chronic pain states. *Drugs* 1993;46:313-340.

27. Sykes N P. Methods of assessment of bowel function in patients with advanced cancer. *Palliat Med* 1990;4:287-292.

28. Bruera E, Suarez-Almazor M, Velasco A, Bertolino M, MacDonald SM, Hanson J. The assessment of constipation in terminal cancer patients admitted to a palliative care unit. *J Pain Symptom Manage* 1994;9:515-519.

29. Barr RG, Levine MD, Wilkinson RH, Mulvihill D. Occult stool retention: A clinical tool for its evaluation in school aged children. *Clin Pediat* 1979;18:674-679.

30. Sykes NP. Methods for clinical research in constipation. In Max M, Lynn J (eds.), *Symptom research: Methods and opportunities. An interactive textbook.* Bethesda: National Institutes of Dental and Craniofacial Research, 2001. Available online at <www.symptomresearch.com/chapter_3/index.htm>.

31. McMillan SC, Williams FA. Validity and reliability of the Constipation Assessment Scale. *Cancer Nurs* 1989;12:183-188.

32. Frank L, Kleinman L, Farup C, Taylor L, Miner P. Psychometric validation of a constipation assessment questionnaire. *Scand J Gastroenterol* 1999;34:870-877.

33. Holdstock D J, Misiewicz J J, Smith T, Rowlands E N. Propulsion (mass movements) in the human colon and its relationship to meals and somatic activity. *Gut* 1970;11:91-99.

34. Muller-Lissner S A. Effect of wheat bran on weight of stool and gastrointestinal transit time: a meta-analysis. *Brit Med J* 1988;296:615-617.

35. Mumford S P. Can high fibre diets improve the bowel function in patients on a radiotherapy ward? In Twycross R G, Lack S A. *Control of alimentary symptoms in far advanced cancer.* Edinburgh: Churchill Livingstone; 1986:183.

36. Ramesh PR, Suresh Kumar K, Rajagopal MR, Balachandran P, Warrier PK. Managing morphine-induced constipation: A controlled comparison of an Ayurvedic formulation and senna. *J Pain Symptom Manage* 1998;16:240-244.

37. Wenk R, Bertolino M, Ochoa J, Cullen C, Bertucelli, Bruera E. Laxative effects of fresh baker's yeast. *J Pain Symptom Manage* 2000;19:163-164.

38. Broide E, Pintov S, Portnoy S, Barg J, Klinowski E, Scapa E. Effectiveness of acupuncture for treatment of childhood constipation. *Digest Dis Sci* 2001;46:1270-1275.

39. Emly M, Cooper S, Vail A. Colonic motility in profoundly disabled people: A comparison of massage and laxative therapy in the management of constipation. *Physiotherapy* 1998;84:178-183.

40. Preece J. Introducing abdominal massage in palliative care for the relief of constipation. *Complement Ther Nurs Midwifery* 2002;5:101-105.

41. Jones MP. Talley NJ. Nuyts G. Dubois D. Lack of objective evidence of efficacy of laxatives in chronic constipation. *Digest Dis Sci* 2002;47:2222-2230.

42. Petticrew M, Watt I, Sheldon T. Systematic review of the effectiveness of laxatives in the elderly. *Health Technol Assess* 1997;1:1-52.

43. Sykes NP. A volunteer model for the comparison of laxatives in opioid-induced constipation. *J Pain Symptom Manage* 1997;11:363-369.

44. NHS Centre for Reviews and Dissemination. Effectiveness of laxatives in adults. *Eff Health Care* 2001;7(1):1-12.

45. Nusko G, Schneider B, Schneider I. Wittekind C. Hahn EG. Anthranoid laxative use is not a risk factor for colorectal neoplasia: Results of a prospective case control study. *Gut* 2000;46:651-655.

46. Nascimbeni R, Donato F, Ghirardi M, Mariani P, Villanacci V, Salerni B. Constipation, anthranoid laxatives, melanosis coli, and colon cancer: A risk assessment using aberrant crypt foci. *Cancer Epidem Biomarker Prev* 2002;11:753-757.

47. Heinicke EA, Kiernan JA. Resistance of myenteric neurons in the rat's colon to depletion by 1,8-dihydroxyanthraquinone. *J Pharm Pharmacol* 1990;42:123-125.

48. Bateman D N, Smith J M. A policy for laxatives. *Brit Med J* 1988;297:1420-1421.

49. Lederle FA, Busch DL, Mattox KM, West MJ, Aske DM. Cost-effective treatment of constipation in the elderly: A randomised double-blind comparison of sorbitol and lactulose. *Amer J Med* 1990;89:597-601.

50. Culbert P, Gillett H, Ferguson A. Highly effective new oral therapy for faecal impaction. *Brit J Gen Pract* 1998;48:1599-1600.

51. Di Palma JA, Smith JR, Cleveland MVB. Overnight efficacy of polyethylene glycol laxative. *Amer J Gastroenterol* 2002;97:1776-1779.

52. Parnaud G., Corpet DE, Gamet-Payrastre L. Cytostatic effect of polyethylene glycol on human colonic adenocarcinoma cells. *Int J Cancer* 2001;92:63-69.

53. Read NW. Motility: Functional diseases. *Curr Opin Gastroen* 1990;6:9-13.

54. Muller-Lissner S A. Treatment of chronic constipation with cisapride and placebo. *Gut* 1987;28:1033-1038.

55. Emmanuel AV, Roy AJ, Nicholls TJ, Kamm MA. Prucalopride, a systemic enterokinetic, for the treatment of constipation. *Aliment Pharmacol Therapeut* 2002;16:1347-1356.

56. Corsetti M. Tack J. Tegaserod: A new 5-HT$_4$ agonist in the treatment of irritable bowel syndrome. *Expert Opin Pharmacother* 2002;3:1211-1218.

57. Hasler W, Heldsinger A, Soudah H, Owyang C. Erythromycin promotes colonic transit in humans: Mediation via motilin receptors. *Gastroenterology* 1990; 98:A358.

58. Bassotti G, Chiaroni G, Vantini I, Morelli A, Whitehead WE. Effect of different doses of erythromycin on colonic motility in patients with slow transit constipation. *Z Gastroenterol* 1998;36:209-213.

59. Ouwehand AC, Lagstrom H, Suomalainen T, Salminen S. Effect of probiotics on constipation, fecal azoreductase activity and fecal mucin content in the elderly. *Ann Nutr Metab* 2002;46:159-162.

60. Ripamonti C, Bruera E. Chronic nausea and vomiting. In Ripamonti C, Bruera E (eds.), *Gastrointestinal symptoms in advanced cancer patients.* Oxford: Oxford University Press; 2002:168-192.

61. Blancquaert JP, LeFebvre RA, Willems JL. Emetic and antiemetic effects of opioids in the dog. *Eur J Pharmacol* 1986;128:143-150.

62. Abbot FK, Mack M, Wolf S. The relation of sustained contraction of the duodenum to nausea and vomiting. *Gastroenterology,* 1952;20:238-248.

63. Twycross RG, Lack SA. *Control of alimentary symptoms in far advanced cancer.* Edinburgh: Churchill Livingstone; 1986:153.

64. Stewart JJ, Weisbrodt NW, Burko TF. Intestinal reverse peristalsis associated with morphine-induced vomiting. In Kosterlitz HW (ed.), *Opiates and endogenous opioid peptides.* Amsterdam: Elsevier; 1976:46-58.

65. Bruera E, MacEachern TJ, Spachynski KA, LeGatt DF, MacDonald RN, Babul N, Harsanyi Z, Darke AC. Comparison of the efficacy, safety and pharmacokinetics of controlled release and immediate release metoclopramide for the management of chronic nausea in patients with advanced cancer. *Cancer* 1994;74: 3204-3211.

66. Critchley P, Plach N, Grantham M, Marshall D, Taniguchi A, Latimer E. Efficacy of haloperidol in the treatment of nausea and vomiting in the palliative patient: A systematic review. *J Pain Symptom Manage* 2001;22:631-634.

67. Twycross RG. The use of low dose levomepromazine (methotrimeprazine) in the management of nausea and vomiting. *Prog Palliat Care* 1997;5:49-53.

68. Passik S, Lundberg J, Kirsh KL, Theobald D, Donaghy K, Holtsclaw E, Coper M, Dugan W. A pilot exploration of the antiemetic activity of olanzepine for the relief of nausea in patients with advanced cancer. *J Pain Symptom Manage* 2002; 23:526-532.

69. Dundee JW, Jones PO. The prevention of analgesic-induced nausea and vomiting by cyclizine. *Brit J Clin Pract* 1968;22:379-382.

70. Walder AD, Aitkenhead AR. A comparison of droperidol and cyclizine in the prevention of postoperative nausea and vomiting associated with patient-controlled analgesia. *Anaesthesia* 1995;50:654-656.

71. Cole RF, Robinson F, Harvey L, Trethowan K, Murdoch V. Successful control of intractable nausea and vomiting requiring combined ondansetron and haloperidol in a patient with advanced cancer. *J Pain Symptom Manage* 1994;9:48-50.

72. Loewen PS. Anti-emetics in development. *Expert Opin Investig Drugs* 2002; 11:801-805.

73. Dundee JW, Chestnutt WN, Ghaly RG, Lynas AGA. Traditional Chinese acupuncture: A potentially useful antiemetic? *Brit Med J* 1986;293:583-584.

74. Lee A, Done ML. The use of non-pharmacologic techniques to prevent postoperative nausea and vomiting: A meta-analysis. *Anesth Analg* 1999;88:1362-1369.

75. Mercadante S, Casuccio A, Groff L, Boffi R, Villari P, Gebbia V, Ripamonti C. Switching form morphine to methadone to improve analgesia and tolerability in cancer patients. A prospective study. *J Clin Oncol* 2001;19:2898-2904.

76. Hunt R, Fazekas B, Thorne D, Brooksbank M. A comparison of subcutaneous morphine and fentanyl in hospice cancer patients. *J Pain Symptom Manage* 1999;18:111-119.

Chapter 6

Opioid Bowel Dysfunction in Acute and Chronic Nonmalignant Pain

Keri L. Fakata
Ashok K. Tuteja
Arthur G. Lipman

INTRODUCTION

Pain is the most common reason that persons enter the health care system and over 50 million Americans report chronic pain annually.[1] There are an estimated 25 million doctor visits for low back pain alone. Approximately 45 percent of Americans seek medical care for a painful condition at some time in their lives.[2] Opioids remain the most effective medications for moderate to severe acute pain and cancer pain, and the usefulness of these drugs as well as the importance of using them when medically indicated is increasingly recognized in chronic nonmalignant pain (CNMP) management.[3,4] Major erosion of quality of life and an estimated $80 billion in lost productivity are attributed to CNMP annually in the United States and it is probable that more aggressive analgesic pharmacotherapy could decrease the huge impact that CNMP has on American society.[2] However, many clinicians hesitate to prescribe opioids and many patients fear taking them due to adverse effects. One of the most common and troublesome of these effects is opioid-induced constipation.

Constipation, per se, is another reason that Americans often seek medical attention. An estimated 2.5 million physician visits per year are due to constipation.[5] Approximately 85 percent of these visits result in recommendations for laxative therapy. The prevalence of constipation in the general community is reported to be as high as 28 percent.[6] Constipation is usually defined by bowel frequency, e.g., fewer than three complete bowel movements in a week. Patients' descriptions of constipation vary widely. They may describe straining, hard stool, a sense of wanting to defecate but being unable to do so, incomplete bowel evacuation, and abdominal discomfort.

There is broad consensus on the importance of using regularly scheduled stimulating laxative regimens for patients taking opioids on a regular schedule for the management of chronic malignant pain.[4,7] This chapter addresses issues associated with opioid-induced constipation in acute pain and CNMP. The impact of opioid bowel dysfunction in acute and CNMP as well as recommendations of currently available laxative therapies are presented with a proposed role for peripheral opioid antagonists in the management of opioid-induced constipation. Exhibit 6.1 lists possible manifestations of opioid bowel dysfunction (OBD).

DIFFERENTIATING PAIN TYPES

A 1986, National Institutes of Health (NIH) consensus conference concluded that pain is not a single entity. In other words, it is useful to consider pain as falling into three major categories: acute pain, chronic pain associated with malignant disease (chronic malignant pain), and chronic pain not associated with malignant disease (chronic nonmalignant pain).[8] Differences among these three types of pain are listed in Table 6.1. Acute pain results from direct tissue damage and

---

EXHIBIT 6.1. Manifestations of opioid bowel dysfunction.

> Abdominal pain
> Abdominal distension
> Nausea/vomiting
> Hard dry stool
> Straining
> Pseudodiarrhea
> Anorexia
> Gastroesophageal reflux disorder

Source: Adapted from Klaschik E, Nauck F, Ostgathe C. Constipation— modern laxative therapy. *Support Care Cancer* 2003;11:679-685.

TABLE 6.1. Differences among acute, chronic malignant, and chronic nonmalignant pain.

Characteristic	Acute	Chronic pain of nonmalignant origin	Chronic pain of malignant origin
Duration	Hours to days resolves as causative insult resolves	Months to years	Unpredictable
Associated pathology	Present	Often none	Usually present
Prognosis	Predictable	Unpredictable	Increasing pain with possibility of disfigurement and fear of dying
Associated problems	Uncommon	Depression, anxiety, secondary gain issues	Many, especially fear of loss of control
Nerve conduction	Rapid	Slow	Slow
Autonomic nervous system involvement	Present	Generally absent	Present or absent
Biological value	High	Low or absent	Low
Social effects	Minimal	Profound	Variable—usually marked
Treatment	Primarily analgesics	Multimodal: often largely physical and behavioral therapy; drugs usually are adjunctive, not primary therapy	Multimodal: drugs usually play a major role

Source: Adapted from Lipman AG. Drug therapy in the management of pain. *Brit J Pharm Pract* 1990;12:22-29.

usually signals underlying pathology. Tissue damage most commonly results from athletic injuries, surgical or medical procedures, and other trauma. The cause of acute pain is not always readily identifiable, for example, acute chest pain may result from myocardial infarction, gastroesophogeal reflux disease, or acute anxiety. Acute pain is usually sharp, shooting, and moderate to severe in intensity.

Sympathetic branch autonomic nervous system stimulation occurs with acute pain and is associated with tachycardia, hypertension, diaphoresis, and mydriasis. The pain usually abates as the tissue insult resolves. If not adequately managed, acute pain can slow healing and promote neuronal plasticity within the nervous system, resulting in chronic pain.

Pain is considered chronic when its duration exceeds the expected healing time or the tissue insult continues due to malignant or nonmalignant ongoing pathology, for example, cancer or arthritis, respectively. Underlying pathology for some chronic pain cannot be identified. This can result from neuronal plasticity, learned pain behavior, or psychogenic pain syndromes. Chronic pain without an identifiable physical cause may be associated with Axis I and II psychiatric diagnoses. Chronic pain encompasses a number of painful nociceptive and neuropathic syndromes, for example, myofascial pain, failed back syndrome, fibromyalgia syndrome. It can be mild to severe, intermittent or constant. In contrast to acute pain, chronic pain is usually not associated with autonomic nervous system (sympathetic branch) activation. Pain behaviors and signs that are common in acute pain patients often are absent in chronic pain patients. The treatment of chronic pain is complex, often requiring a multimodal approach by an interdisciplinary treatment program with input from physicians, nurses, physical therapists, psychologists, and clinical pharmacists who have specialized pain management training and experience.

OPIOID BOWEL DYSFUNCTION IN ACUTE PAIN

Opioids frequently cause constipation, but the prevalence of this problem and the impact of opioid pharmacotherapy have not been defined in acute pain patients. Most studies of opioid-induced constipation have been done in cancer and palliative care patients, as discussed in the preceding chapters.

An evaluation of patient-controlled analgesia (PCA) in 915 postoperative patients revealed a 22 percent prevalence of constipation.[9] It is probable that constipation is more prevalent with oral than parenteral opioid therapy. This hypothesis is supported by the observation that oral naloxone, a μ opioid antagonist, can reverse opioid-induced constipation (presumably due to local enteric effects) in some patients without reversing analgesia (central systemic effects) in patients taking oral opioids for acute pain due to the direct exposure to the gastrointestinal tract. The gut is highly sensitive to local effects of opioids; it takes more opioid to achieve analgesia than to produce constipation. Animal studies in rats and mice have indicated that 4 times more morphine is required to achieve analgesia than constipation by the subcutaneous route, and 20 times more by the oral route.[10] It is probable that constipation is more prevalent with oral than parenteral opioid therapy due to direct contact with gut opioid receptors. Oral opioids are commonly used to treat acute pain. Loperamide is an opioid agonist that is not well absorbed from the GI tract and is used for its constipating effects to treat diarrhea. Alvimopan is an investigational oral peripheral opioid antagonist that has only 0.03 percent oral bioavailability. Earlier studies have demonstrated that this agent may reverse opioid bowel dysfunction.[11] Opioid-induced constipation appears to be both a local and systemic effect. The development of peripheral opioid antagonists has helped to differentiate between a central and peripheral mediation in OBD with peripheral being more dominant. OBD is also reported as a common early side effect in patients on intrathecal opioids.[12] The intrathecal route limits systemic absorption of opioid, and central mediated OBD is demonstrated; however systemic absorption may be adequate enough to demonstrate peripheral OBD. Route of administration may impact OBD (oral > intravenous ≥ transdermal ≥ epidural > intrathecal).

Opioid-induced constipation may add to the discomfort experienced by patients with acute pain as might opioid-induced nausea and vomiting. Many postoperative patients are unable to ingest anything by mouth following their surgery. Rectal preparations that might be used are discussed later in the chapter. Constipation is associated with nausea, vomiting, abdominal distension, and pain. Patients in acute pain who are receiving opioids should also receive an appropriate bowel regimen to prevent opioid-induced constipation. Principles of laxative therapy for the treatment of opioid-induced constipation are addressed later in this chapter.

OPIOID BOWEL DYSFUNCTION IN CHRONIC NONMALIGNANT PAIN

The prevalence and etiology of constipation in CNMP patients who receive chronic opioid therapy has not been well characterized. A telephone survey addressing opioid treatment and bowel habits of 76 CNMP patients was reported in abstract form at the 1999 American Pain Society meeting and the results of that survey were compared to a separate national survey of 10,018 nonopioid subjects. Over 40 percent of subjects taking opioids reported fewer than three bowel movements in a week compared to fewer than 8 percent of the subjects in national survey. Other symptoms of constipation such as incomplete bowel movements, straining, and hard stools were reported three to four times more frequently by respondents taking opioids than those not taking the drugs.[13] Moulin et al. reported a 46 percent incidence of constipation in 46 patients treated for 9 weeks with morphine for CNMP.[14]

Transdermal fentanyl has been reported to have less constipating effect than other opioids when used in CNMP management. One study of transdermal fentanyl for the treatment of chronic low back pain documented a 46 percent occurrence of constipation regardless of dose.[15] A later study that compared transdermal fentanyl to continuous-release (CR) morphine for CNMP documented a 16 percent incidence of constipation for the fentanyl treatment group and 22 percent for the morphine group. A bowel questionnaire demonstrated significant reduction in constipation (48 percent morphine CR versus 29 percent fentanyl, $p < 0.001$). An additional trial that evaluated the long-term safety and efficacy of transdermal fentanyl in CNMP reported that constipation occurred either as possible or definite treatment-related adverse event in 19 percent of patients.[16]

A major shortcoming of several published studies of opioid-induced constipation is the failure of the investigators to use standardized criteria for defining constipation. Different patients have varied perception of symptoms of constipation, and not using precise criteria can alter reports of constipation prevalence. A recent study evaluated the prevalence of OBD, risk factors, health care utilization, and its association with pain control and health-related quality of life (HRQoL) by administrating a validated modified bowel disease questionnaire that included the Rome criteria for functional bowel disorders, and the Treatment Outcomes in Pain Survey (TOPS, a validated, augmented SF-36 to measure pain-related HRQoL) in CNMP.[17-19] Constipation was reported by 53 percent of subjects, fewer than three bowel movements per week and incomplete evacuation were reported by 35 percent, straining by 43 percent, hard stool by 47 percent, and the need for digital evacuation was reported by 21 percent. Prevalence of constipation and its symptoms were equally common in males and females. This study also demonstrated that constipation in patients on opioids is not associated with age, marital status, education level, smoking, or alcohol consumption. No association was found between dose of opioids and prevalence of constipation.[20] Unexpectedly, diarrhea was reported by 21 percent of subjects in this study, and the presence of constipation was not associated with pain symptoms or the total pain experience. Neither the patients' satisfaction nor HRQoL measures were affected by constipation. Confounding factors to consider when evaluating CNMP patients with OBD are polypharmacy, psychosocial issues, and concomitant functional bowel disorders, such as irritable bowel syndrome (IBS). Irritable bowel syndrome can present with diarrhea, constipation, or combination of the two. Opioids may normalize loose bowel movements or exacerbate constipation in a CNMP patient with IBS.

IS OPIOID BOWEL DYSFUNCTION PROPERLY ADDRESSED IN THESE POPULATIONS?

Only a very limited literature evaluates the prevalence and etiology of OBD in pain patients. Most commonly held beliefs about constipation and its prevention and management are based on anecdotes, not evidence, and recent studies have proven several of these common beliefs to be incorrect. Limited health care staffing and resources, as well as dramatically shortened lengths of hospital stay following surgery, have decreased clinicians' ability to monitor outcomes of postoperative patients' opioid use. OBD often is not discussed during outpatient emergency department visits or with patients who go to emergency care centers and are given opioids for work-related injuries.

Not infrequently, patients have to make less than well-informed decisions in the laxative aisles of their local pharmacies. Most patient counseling about opioids emphasizes acute effects such as sedation, risks of driving or operating machinery, and gastrointestinal (GI) upset. A pharmacy-based intervention study of laxative prescribing in patients started on opioids revealed that only 31 percent of patients received a concurrent laxative prescription with opioids.[21] In the previously mentioned study of 76 CNMP patients receiving opioids, 80 percent of those patients were taking laxatives, of whom only 46 percent reported successful laxation at least half of the time.[13] Even when OBD is addressed and laxatives are used, some patients do not experience adequate relief of opioid-induced constipation.

CURRENT TREATMENT OPTIONS
FOR OPIOID BOWEL DYSFUNCTION

Both nonpharmacological and pharmacological approaches to the treatment of opioid-induced constipation should be used for optimal management. Most pharmacological options for the treatment of OBD are available over the counter, in other words, without a prescription. All patients receiving more than occasional doses of opioids should be counseled about appropriate use of an over-the-counter bowel regimen. Besides opioids, any other associated causes of constipation should be recognized, especially difficulty reaching the bathroom, mechanical bowel obstruction, neurological disorders, metabolic disorder, and other associated constipating drugs. The constipation may not be manageable until those confounding factors are addressed effectively. Nonpharmacologic approaches may help prevent and manage OBD, but often they are not adequate. Many patients require the combination of nonpharmacological and pharmacological techniques to properly manage OBD.

Patient Education

Clinicians should educate patients about normal bowel habits, diet, fluid intake, and exercise. Patients who believe that bowels must move every day should be informed that a bowel movement every other day or sometimes every third day is not abnormal. Patients who miss meals should be encouraged to eat more regularly. Increased fluid intake and physical activity are generally recommended for the management of constipation. However, patients who ingest adequate fluid and are well hydrated generally do not benefit from increasing fluid intake because further increases in fluid are reabsorbed in the intestines.[22] Immobility increases the risk of OBD complications ranging from symptomatic constipation to bowel obstruction. This may be problematic for some pain patients because many painful disorders for which opioid therapy is indicated make activity difficult, if not impossible. Increased physical activity does not seem to benefit patients who are normally active.[23,24] Colonic mass movements follow a circadian pattern, with decrease in colonic propulsive activity at night and steep increase after meals, especially on awakening in the morning.[25] Caffeinated coffee enhances the gastrocolonic response, increases colonic motility, and induces fluid secretion in small intestine.[26,27] Many patients with constipation may be managed with a regular bowel regimen practiced over an adequate amount of time,[28] a higher fiber diet, and spending 15 to 20 minutes on the toilet after breakfast and coffee.

Nonprescription Options for Opioid Bowel Dysfunction

Increase Dietary Fiber

In general, Americans do not ingest sufficient dietary fiber. We consume an average of 5 to 14 grams a day, far below the 20 to 35 grams recommended by the American Dietetic Association.[29] Dietary fiber intake can be increased by eating more fruits and vegetables, whole grain breads, and cereals. Patients should not attempt to increase fiber in their diet if they are immobile or do not have adequate fluid intake. Opioids induce constipation by inhibiting the secretory processes and decreasing motility of the bowel. The combination of immobility and poor fluid intake puts patient at risk of bowel obstruction. The evidence does not support efficacy of increased dietary fiber in patients already taking the recommended amounts, but this approach may be useful in patients who ingest little fiber. Patients' compliance with fiber can be improved by increasing fiber intake gradually over a period of one to two weeks. Many patients ingesting increased fiber complain of flatulence and bloating secondary to colonic fermentation of unabsorbed fiber.[17]

Pharmacological Options for Prevention and Treatment of Opioid Bowel Dysfunction

There are five classes of nonprescription laxatives that are not necessarily interchangeable. There have been a few systematic reviews done in laxative use and treatment of chronic constipation in adults. Laxatives are generally associated with increased bowel movement frequency and improvement of symptoms of constipation. There is little evidence that one laxative is better than another in the general population.[5,30] However the mechanisms of action of these drugs suggest types of constipation of which some classes may be better than others, and some types of constipation for which certain laxatives are not appropriate, for example, opioid-induced constipation. Most of the few comparative laxative studies that have been published are small and methodologically flawed. The treatment and prevention of opioid-induced constipation may require a combination of more than one class of laxatives. The most common regimen for opioid-induced constipation is a stimulating laxative combined with a stool softener. However, opioid-induced constipation may not respond adequately to this therapy, necessitating a more aggressive approach.

It is important to tailor laxative regimens to the individual patient. For example, in a spinal cord injury patient who no longer has a cough reflex, the risk of aspiration necessitates avoiding laxatives such as lactulose that often cause nausea and vomiting. Table 6.2 lists some specific information on the various laxatives classes.

Stool Softeners

Stool softeners simply increase the hydration of stool; they do not stimulate bowel evacuation. The mechanism of action of stool softeners involves better mixing of water into the stool from surfactant effects of the drugs and may also include secretion of isotonic fluid from the proximal intestine, increasing fluid content of the forming stool. It is important to recognize that stool softeners are not laxatives per se. These agents can help facilitate bowel evacuation when hard, dry stools occur in the presence of sufficient peristaltic propulsion. However, in the presence of decreased peristalsis, as is the case with opioid therapy, stool softeners alone usually provide no benefit—because the softened stool sits in the bowel, which has decreased

TABLE 6.2. Some commonly used laxative preparations.

Type	Product	Dosage	Time	Side effects	Comments
Lubricant	Petrolatum	15-45 mL at bedtime	6-8 h oral	Anal incontinence Anal irritation	Prolonged use decreases absorption of fat-soluble vitamins ADEK
	Mineral oil (Fleet Enema)	118 mL rectal	15-30 min	Oil leakage from	Avoid in patients with aspiration risk (lipid pneumonia) Avoid taking with meal, may delay gastric emptying Separate other medications by 2 h
Osmotic laxatives	Sodium phosphate (Fleet Enema; Fleet Phospo Soda)	100 mL/enema 20-30 mL mixed in half glass of cold water			Up to 20% of oral dose may be absorbed systemically Avoid in renal dysfunction Use only when evacuation needed
	Glycerin	3 g rectally	30 min	Rectal irritation	Rare
Saline	Magnesium citrate	150-300 mL po	30 min-3 h oral	Abdominal cramping	Hypermagnesia Hyperphosphotemia Hypocalcemia
	Magnesium hydroxide (Phillips', Milk of Magnesia)	15-40 mL HS	2-5 min rectal	Excessive diuresis Nausea/vomiting Dehydration	Contraindications Ileostomy Colostomy Dehydration Congestive heart failure
	Magnesium sulfate (Epsom salts)	10-15 g dissolved in fluid			Potential for significant drug interactions, e.g., Warfarin, digoxin, phenothiazines

TABLE 6.2 (continued)

Type	Product	Dosage	Time	Side effects	Comments
Isotonic laxative	Polyethylene glycol	17 g/day dissolved in 8 oz of fluid	Initial 2-4 days Then 24 h	Abdominal fullness Bloating Flatulence Diarrhea	Must take necessary amount of fluid Well tolerated
Saccharine laxatives	Lactulose (Enulose) Sorbitol	15-45 mL t.i.d. to q.i.d, max 40 mg/day or 60 mL	2-48 h	Bloating Cramping Nausea/vomiting Diarrhea Epigastric pain Flatulence	Electrolyte imbalance Excessive gas May give lactulose or sorbitol as a retention enema
Stimulant laxatives					
Anthranoids	Senna	2 tabs q.i.d. to 4 tabs b.i.d. Dosage form: Tablet Tea Liquid Concentrate	8-12 h	Abdominal cramping Griping Flatulence Diarrhea	Use standardized senna glycosides Pseudomelanous coli (reversible) Causes cathartic colon (unproven)

112

Diphenyl methane	Bisacodyl	10 to 30 mg Suppository 10 mg	6-10 h 15-60 min	Abdominal cramping Flatulence Diarrhea Malabsorption Electrolyte disturbances	Rectal burning with daily use of suppository Incontinence of bowel Enteric-coated tablets (do not crush)
Miscellaneous	Castrol oil	15-60 mL	2-6 h	Abdominal cramping Flatulence Diarrhea Malabsorption Electrolyte disturbances	Most effective when administered on an empty stomach Not very palatable

Sources: Pappagallo M. Incidence, prevalence, and management of opioid bowel dysfunction. *Am J Surg* 2001;182:11S-18S; Curry Jr CE, Butler DM, Constipation. In Allen Jr LV, Bernardi RR, DeSimone II EM, Engle JP, Popovich NG, Monroe-Rosenthal W, Tietze KJ (ed.), *Handbook of nonprescription drugs*, 12 ed. Washington, DC: American Pharmaceutical Association; 2000:273-300.

peristaltic activity due to the opioid, and the intestines simply re-absorb water making the stool hard and dry. Docusate sodium is a stool softener commonly used in combination with a stimulant laxative, for example, senna, bisacodyl, for the prevention and treatment of opioid-induced constipation. Stool softeners alone may be agents of choice for patients with hard, dry stools who do not have difficulty initiating bowel movements but experience discomfort or inability to evacuate due to hardness of the stool.

Bulk Producers

Bulk-producing laxatives are indigestible hydrophilic colloids such as psyllium and methylcellulose. They absorb water to produce bulk that distends the colon. This in turn stimulates peristalsis. Bulk laxatives are not appropriate for patients with impaired peristalsis, in other words, those with opioid induced constipation, because the stretching of a colon that cannot respond with peristalsis can cause painful, colicky symptoms.

If patients do not maintain adequate fluid intake, bulk producers can worsen constipation and increase the risk for bowel obstruction. These agents should absolutely be avoided in patients that are fluid restricted, confined to bed, or have signs of partial obstruction.

Bulk producers are often the laxatives of choice for "occasional constipation" in normal, otherwise healthy patients.

Lubricants

Laxatives that lubricate the intestinal track, especially the rectum, can be useful for patients with hemorrhoids, anal fissures, or who otherwise have difficulty passing stool due to mechanical limitations. Common examples are mineral oil taken either orally or via enema and glycerin suppositories. Thus rectal administration of an enema or suppository also has some mechanical stimulatory action. Lubricants are most commonly used as adjuncts to other laxatives. A commercially available combination of mineral oil and milk of magnesia is marketed as Haley's M-O.

Osmotic Laxatives

Osmotic laxatives are hypertonic agents that draw extralumenal water into the colon. They include saline laxatives such as magnesium hydroxide (milk of magnesia) and sodium phosphate (phospho soda). Both oral and rectal forms (e.g., Fleet Enema) are available. Salts in the saline laxatives can be absorbed systemically, and electrolyte imbalances can occur if the patient is not well hydrated. Patients who are at risk from saline cathartics include those with congestive heart failure, cirrhosis, and renal insufficiency. Electrolyte imbalance can also occur due to dehydration resulting from overuse of the saline laxative. To overcome this effect of saline laxatives, polyethylene glycol can be combined with an isoosmotic electrolyte solution. This type of formulation is commonly used for colonoscopy bowel preparations. MiraLax is a polyethylene glycol preparation used for treatment of chronic constipation. Polyethylene glycol holds water in the colon. It is tolerated well and is becoming popular in the management of OBD in patients that can tolerate the fluid requirement.[31]

Other osmotic laxatives include sorbitol and lactulose. Sorbitol is a polyhydric alcohol that reduces the pH of the stool and also softens the stool. A disadvantage of sorbitol is its very sweet taste. Lactulose is a synthetic disaccharide that is broken down by bacteria in the colon to yield organic acids and carbon dioxide to lower the pH and soften the stool. Lactulose also is unpalatable for many patients, often more so than sorbitol. Both of these sugars are also used for ammonium ion trapping in hepatic encephalitis. For aggressive bowel program these agents are usually given orally every two hours until a bowel movement occurs. Lactulose commonly causes nausea and vomiting when used in this way; sorbitol is better tolerated. These two laxatives are most commonly used for patients who have failed with combined stool softener and stimulant laxative for the treatment of opioid-induced constipation.

The milder saline osmotic laxatives are commonly used as alternatives to bulk producers for occasional constipation in otherwise healthy patients.

Stimulant Laxatives

Stimulants increase bowel evacuation by irritating sensory nerve endings to initiate the parasympathetic reflex that increases peristalsis. Senna (standardized senna concentrate, pure sennosides) is an anthraquinone laxative derived from plants that is commonly used in combination with a stool softener for treatment and prevention of opioid-induced constipation. Senna is thought to directly stimulate intestinal mucosal sensory nerve endings activating the parasympathetic plexus. This produces increased motility and may also stimulate prostaglandin synthesis. Senna is not thought to interrupt usual patterns of defecation. Anthranoids are the most studied laxative in terms of drug safety. The pure senna glycosides are preferred over crude senna. Anthranoids can cause deposition of dark brown granular pigment in the colonic mucosa called melanosis coli. The clinical significance of melanosis coli, apart from its association with anthracene laxatives abuse, is uncertain. Pigmentation is reversible upon discontinuation.[32] Bisacodyl is another commonly used stimulating laxative that also causes structural damage to surface epithelial cells and possibly submucosal nerves. There is no clear evidence that stimulant laxatives cause damage to enteric nerve endings and smooth muscle cells within the colon. Evidence linking stimulant laxative use to cathartic colon and increased risk of colon cancer is conflicting.[33] However these issues should be taken into consideration when using a stimulant laxative on a chronic basis.

Overuse of any stimulant laxatives can reduce colonic tone, making the patient dependent on the laxatives for defecation. This cautionary statement has deterred many physicians from recommending stimulant laxatives for their patients with OBD. It is important to differentiate between safe and effective use of stimulant laxatives for chronic use and overuse. Pain patients on chronic opioid therapy may need prolonged laxative therapy to overcome opioid-induced constipation, but daily use of a stimulant may not be needed. The goal for the chronic pain patient is to try to achieve a bowel movement every other day to every third day. Fluid and electrolyte complications also can occur with prolonged stimulant laxative use.

Castor oil is a stimulant laxative but is often mistaken to be a lubricant similar to mineral oil. Castor oil is an irritant, not a lubricant. The oil is degraded to ricinoleic acid that acts as a direct irritant to the gastrointestinal tract, stimulating peristalsis. Castor oil can cause cramping and is toxic in overdose. It is rarely used nowadays due to intolerable side effects. Several other plant derivative stimulating laxatives are available, for example, cascara sagrada. Most of these "natural" agents are very irritating and frequently cause cramping and griping.

Phenolphthalein was a commonly used laxative found in Ex-Lax and numerous other nonprescription formulations until it was shown to be carcinogenic and removed from the market in the 1990s. Over-the-counter laxatives that used to contain phenolphthalein now contain bisacodyl or another stimulant in place of phenolphthalein.[34] Stimulants often are the laxatives of choice for constipation induced by opioids or anticholinergic agents, but they are not preferred for use in patients with normal peristaltic tone.

Opioid Antagonists

Opioid-induced constipation is believed to be due largely to activation of μ opioid receptors in the colon, resulting in markedly decreased peristalsis (as discussed in *Section I: Basic Concepts in Opioid Bowel Dysfunction*). Parenteral opioid antagonists, for example, naloxone, are poorly absorbed from the gastrointestinal tract and have been used orally to help reverse opioid-induced constipation. Results of these trials have been mixed, but some patients have experienced dangerous reversal of their opioid analgesia, presumably due to systemic absorption. Absorption of oral opioid antagonists may increase in patients with advanced diseases due to loss of integrity of their intestines secondary to multiorgan disease.

Methylnaltrexone and alvimopan are investigational, peripherally acting opioid antagonists that were being studied clinically at the time of this writing for opioid-induced constipation. They are discussed in Chapters 10 and 11 of this book. Methylnaltrexone is being investigated as a subcutaneous injection for opioid-induced constipation in terminally ill patients. In the absence of bowel obstruction, this relatively fast-acting agent may be beneficial for symptomatic constipation.[10] Alvimopan is in oral dosage form that may take just as long as the standard laxative regimens to produce a bowel movement but may be more reliable in producing a bowel movement due to its specific mechanism of action. These agents will most probably be far more expensive than laxative regimens if and when they become commercially available. They should most likely be reserved for OBD cases that are not responsive to standard laxative regimens. It is not yet known if peripheral opioid antagonists will become less effective if they are overused. Theoretically, they should have lower risk of inducing atonic bowel or for patients to become dependent on them for bowel function.

Opioids are presumed to cause constipation by decreasing gastrointestinal motility and increasing fluid absorption. The management described here related to slow transit constipation. If patients do not respond to this regimen and if obstructive constipation is suspected, colon transit and anorectal physiological testing may be indicated. The demonstration of abnormal pelvic floor coordination and abnormal psychological profiles in these patients would suggest that bowel disorder may be amenable to behavioral treatment. Biofeedback results in decreased straining and even an improved transit time in patients with constipation.[18]

CONCLUSION

The prevalence of OBD in acute and chronic pain patients receiving opioids has not been well characterized, but research into this issue is ongoing. Most available data are from studies in cancer and palliative care patients. Opioids often cause constipation, and symptomatic opioid-induced constipation may affect the quality of pain control achieved by patients taking those drugs. Many patients respond adequately to a standard bowel regimen, but others do not. Risk factors associated with increased complication are not yet known. More predictable and effective bowel regimens are needed in such cases to manage symptomatic OBD.

Acute pain and CNMP are very common and too often are not well managed. Opioid-induced constipation is an often overlooked component of the discomfort that patients suffer. Acute pain patients frequently receive opioids for pain associated with surgery, trauma, and medical procedures. Opioids are being used increasingly in a broad range of CNMP syndromes as well. Clinicians should maintain a relatively high index of suspicion about opioid-induced constipation for all patients receiving opioids and should prevent and manage this iatrogenic complication whenever needed.

NOTES

1. Chronic pain in America: Road blocks to relief. Roper Starch World Wide Inc. 1999. Available online at <http://www.ampainsoc.org/whatsnew/summary2_road. htm>.

2. Bonica J. *The management of pain,* 2nd ed. Philadelphia: Lea and Febiger; 1990.

3. Model guidelines for the use of controlled substances for the treatment of pain. *Federation of State Medical Boards.* 1998. Available online at <http://www.fsmb.org/Policy%20Documents%20and%20White%20Papers/model_pain_guidelines.htm>. Accessed Decemeber 19th, 2003.

4. Jacox A, Carr DB, Payne R, Berde CB, Breitbart W, Cain JM, Chapman CR, Cleeland CS, Ferrell BR, Finley RS, et al. *Managment of cancer pain. Clinical practice guideline.* Vol AHCPR Publication Number 94-0592. Rockville, MD: Agency for Healthcare Policy and Research; 1994.

5. Tramonte SM, Brand MB, Mulrow CD, Amato MG, O'Keefe ME, Ramirez G. The treatment of chronic constipation in adults: A systematic review. *J Gen Intern Med* 1997;12:15-24.

6. Locke GR III, Pemberton JH, Phillips SF. AGA technical review on constipation. *Gastroenterology* 2000;119:1766-1778.

7. American Pain Society. *Principles of analgesic use in the treatment of acute pain and chronic cancer pain,* 5th ed. Glenview, IL: American Pain Society; 2003.

8. The integrated approach to the management of pain. *NIH Consensus Statement* May 19-21, 1986;6:1-8.

9. Karci A, Tasdogen A, Erkin Y, Sahinoz B, Kara H, Elar Z. Evaluation of quality in patient-controlled analgesia provided by an acute pain service. *Eur Surg Res* 2003;35:363-371.

10. Yuan CS FJ. Methylnaltrexone: Investigation of clinical applications. *Drug Development Research* 2000;50:133-141.

11. Schmidt WK. Alvimopan (ADL 8-2698) is a novel peripheral opioid antagonist. *Am J Surg* 2001;182:27S-38S.

12. Paice JA, Winkelmuller W, Burchiel K, Racz GB, Prager JP. Clinical realities and economic considerations: Efficacy of intrathecal pain therapy. *J Pain Symptom Manage* 1997;14:S14-S26.

13. Pappagallo M. Incidence, prevalence, and management of opioid bowel dysfunction. *Am J Surg* 2001;182:11S-18S.

14. Moulin DE, Iezzi A, Amireh R, Sharpe WK, Boyd D, Merskey H. Randomised trial of oral morphine for chronic non-cancer pain. *Lancet* 1996;347:143-147.

15. Simpson RK Jr, Edmondson EA, Constant CF, Collier C. Transdermal fentanyl as treatment for chronic low back pain. *J Pain Symptom Manage* 1997;14:218-224.

16. Milligan K, Lanteri-Minet M, Borchert K, Helmers H, Donald R, Kress HG, Adriaensen H, Mowin D, Jarvimaki V, Haazen L. Evaluation of long-term efficacy and safety of transdermal fentanyl in the treatment of chronic noncancer pain. *J Pain* 2001;2:197-204.

17. Voderholzer WA, Schatke W, Muhldorfer BE, Klauser AG, Birkner B, Muller-Lissner SA. Clinical response to dietary fiber treatment of chronic constipation. *Am J Gastroenterol* 1997;92:95-98.

18. Koutsomanis D, Lennard-Jones JE, Roy AJ, Kamm MA. Controlled randomised trial of visual biofeedback versus muscle training without a visual display for intractable constipation. *Gut* 1995;37:95-99.

19. Rogers WH, Wittnik H, Wagner A, Cynn D, Carr DB. Assessing individual outcomes during outpatient multidisiplinary chronic pain treatment by means of an augmented SF-36. *Pain Medicine* 2000;1:44-54.

20. Fakata K, Tuteja A, Lipman A, Ho M. Opioid-induced constipation: A survey of prevalence and risk factors in chronic non-malignant pain. The 2nd Joint Scientific Meeting of APS and CPS in Vancouver, BC, Canada. May 7-9, 2004: *J Pain* 2004;5(3)Suppl:545.

21. Bouvy ML, Buurma H, Egberts TC. Laxative prescribing in relation to opioid use and the influence of pharmacy-based intervention. *J Clin Pharm Ther* 2002; 27:107-110.

22. Young RJ, Beerman LE, Vanderhoof JA. Increasing oral fluids in chronic constipation in children. *Gastroenterol Nurs* 1998;21:156-161.

23. Tuteja AK, Joos SK, Talley NJ, Woehl J, Hickam DH. Association between constipation and physical activity in a population of employed adults. *Gastroenterol* 2001; 120: Supp 1, A 230. Paper presented at American Gastroenterology Association, 2001, Atlanta, GA.

24. Meshkinpour H, Selod S, Movahedi H, Nami N, James N, Wilson A. Effects of regular exercise in management of chronic idiopathic constipation. *Dig Dis Sci* 1998;43:2379-2383.

25. Bassotti G, Gaburri M, Imbimbo BP, Rossi L, Farroni F, Pelli MA, Morelli A. Colonic mass movements in idiopathic chronic constipation. *Gut* 1988;29:1173-1179.

26. Rao SS, Welcher K, Zimmerman B, Stumbo P. Is coffee a colonic stimulant? *Eur J Gastroenterol Hepato* 1998;10:113-118.

27. Wald A, Back C, Bayless TM. Effect of caffeine on the human small intestine: Is coffee a colonic stimulant? *Gastroenterology* 1976;71:738-742.

28. Karam SE, Nies DM. Student/staff collaboration: A pilot bowel management program. *J Gerontol Nurs* 1994;20:32-40.

29. National Digestive Diseases Information Clearinghouse. Constipation. Available online at <http://digestive.niddk.nih.gov/ddiseases/pubs/constipation/index.htm>.

30. Petticrew M, Rodgers M, Booth A. Effectiveness of laxatives in adults. *Qual Health Care* 2001;10:268-273.

31. Klaschik E, Nauck F, Ostgathe C. Constipation-modern laxative therapy. *Support Care Cancer* 2003;11:679-685.

32. Hallmann F. Toxicity of commonly used laxatives. *Med Sci Monit* 2000; 6:618-628.

33. Wald A. Is chronic use of stimulant laxatives harmful to the colon? *J Clin Gastroenterol.* 2003;36:386-389.

34. National Toxicology Program. Toxicology and carcinogenesis studies of phenolphthalein (CAS No. 77-09-8) in F344/N Rats and B6C3F1 Mice (Feed Studies): National Toxicol Program Tech Report Series No 465, November 1996. Available online at: <http://ntp.niehs.nih.gov/ntp/htdocs/LT_rpts/tr465.pdf>.

Chapter 7

Postoperative Bowel Dysfunction

Cormac Fahy
Tong J. Gan

INTRODUCTION

Postoperative ileus (POI) is defined as an impairment of gastrointestinal mobility after abdominal or other surgery, and is characterized by abdominal distension, lack of bowel sounds, accumulation of gas and fluids in the bowel, and delayed passage of flatus and defecation.[1] Bowel dysfunction postoperatively is often regarded as a normal and inevitable response to laparotomy and other surgical procedures.[2] This is generally accepted to last three to five days postoperatively and is followed by the passage of flatus marking the resumption of peristalsis. Postoperative ileus is a self-limiting functional motility disorder, and is distinguished from mechanical bowel obstruction. Recovery from ileus occurs in a stepwise manner: initial small intestinal motor activity, then gastric motor activity, followed by resumption of colonic motor activity (three to five days).[3]

In the current climate of health care cost minimization, reducing the amount of time a patient spends in the hospital is an important part of health care planning. A postoperative stay after laparotomy ranges from three to ten days depending on the procedure and associated morbidity.[4] Not only on a financial level does this play a significant role, it also leads to delayed mobilization, reduced absorption of medications and food, increased risk of nausea and vomiting, decreased patient satisfaction, and increased risk of infectious and pulmonary complications.[2]

The consequences of bowel dysfunction postoperatively are far-reaching and have many different causes. It is beholden to anesthesiologists and surgeons to find ways of reducing the duration and severity of postoperative ileus for financial, health, and human interests. As opioids play an important role in postoperative bowel dysfunction, methods to minimize their effect either by cotreatment with other agents or minimizing opiate use are an essential component of therapy. The term *multimodal approach* is often applied to management of postoperative ileus, which means attention to surgical technique, perioperative fluids, and enteral nutrition, as well as minimizing the gastrointestinal effects of opiates.

PATHOGENESIS OF POSTOPERATIVE ILEUS

Normal motility in the gastrointestinal tract is dependent on interaction among a number of factors. These include the enteric nervous system, the central nervous system, hormones, and local factors. In addition, motility of the stomach and small intestine is dependent on whether one is in the fasting or fed state. Fasting bowel motility is dependent on the migrating motor complex (MMC) first described by Szurszewski.[5] When fed, motility is governed by a variety of ungrouped low amplitude contractions whose duration and intensity depend on the amount and nature of food ingested. In contrast, the activity in the colon differs both in structure and function to the rest of the bowel. It does not act as a single unit but motility occurs in three ways: oscillatory activity, superimposed spikes, and an unrelated continuous electrical response, which propels contents distally.[6]

Following surgery the normal electrical activity in the gut is impaired. In the stomach, gastric spike and slow wave activity is irregular and, when fasted, the only thing propelling contents is the MMC. In the colon, the three forms of activity are impaired, of which the continuous electrical response is the last to return. However, the onset of electrical activity does not necessarily coincide with the return of normal function.

Why gastrointestinal function is disturbed following surgery is the product of a number of interacting factors outlined in Table 7.1.[6]

Under normal circumstances, the balance between excitatory parasympathetic input and inhibitory sympathetic input ensure normal bowel motility. Experimental studies on rats have shown that reserpine, an adrenergic inhibitor, completely reverses the inhibition to transit of luminal contents caused by laparotomy and partially reverses the inhibition caused by laparotomy and intestinal manipula-

TABLE 7.1. Mechanisms involved in postoperative ileus.

Mechanism	Factors involved
Autonomic nervous system	Sympathetic inhibitory pathways
Enteric nervous system	Substance P, nitric oxide
Hormones and neuropeptides	VIP, CGRP, corticotropin-releasing factor ligands
Inflammation	Macrophage and neutrophil infiltration, cytokines, other mediators
Anesthesia	General anaesthetics
Narcotic analgesics	Opioids

Source: Luckey A, Livingston E, Tache Y. Mechanisms and treatment of postoperative ileus. *Arch Surg* 2003;138:206-214. Copyright © 2003, American Medical Association. All rights reserved.

tion.[7] It has been suggested that hyperactivity of adrenergic neurons activates α_2 adrenoceptors on cholinergic neurons, which leads to a reduction in acetylcholine, with resulting reduction in intestinal motility.[8] Chemical sympathectomy with 6-hydroxydopamine ablates small bowel postoperative ileus and delayed gastric emptying in rats.[9] The inability of sympathetic inhibition to completely resolve postoperative ileus suggests that other mechanisms also contribute.

Local neurotransmitters such as vasoactive intestinal polypeptide (VIP) and substance P both appear to have roles in the development of postoperative ileus.[6] Animal studies have indicated that VIP increases inhibitory input to gastric cholinergic neurons, creating a decrease in antral and pyloric activity.[10] Permanent degeneration of unmyelinated neurons in newborn rats with capsaicin reduced the amount of ileus otherwise produced by iodine.[11]

The most predominant noncholinergic nonadrenergic neurotransmitter in the gastrointestinal tract with an inhibitory role is nitric oxide (NO). Administration of a nitric oxide synthase inhibitor L-NOARG to rats reverses the immotility caused by bowel manipulation.[7] This is postulated to be a constitutive rather than inducible nitric oxide.[7,12]

Administration of calcitonin gene-related peptide (CGRP) antagonists has been shown to partially inhibit postoperative gastric ileus in rats.[6,13] As CGRP is present in visceral afferent neurons and acts on peripheral receptors to delay gastric emptying and gastrointestinal activity,[13,14] it is postulated that abdominal procedures may cause the release of CGRP and so inhibit bowel motility.[6]

The release of endogenous opioids following the trauma of abdominal surgery may have a role in the development of postoperative ileus. In animal studies, infusion of encephalin, a potent opioid receptor agonist, inhibits gastric motility and increases pyloric tone. However, in the context of exogenous opioids given for postoperative pain, their contribution may be minimal.[8,15-17]

Activation of the neurohormonal stress response is a consequence of surgery and anesthesia. A major component of this response is the release of corticotrophin-releasing factor (CRF) from the hypothalamus and related peptides. Peripheral administration of CRF delays gastric emptying in experimental animals and the parenteral injection of a CRF antagonist, α-helical CRF_{9-41}, partially prevents postoperative gastric ileus in rats.[18-20] This suggests a role for CRF in the development of postoperative bowel dysfunction (Figure 7.1).

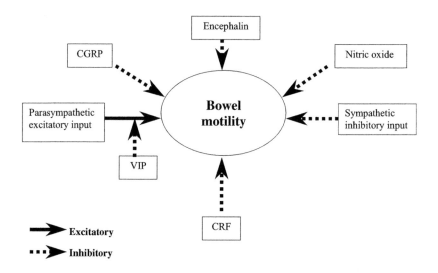

FIGURE 7.1. Physiological factors affecting bowel motility. CGRP = calcitonin gene-related peptide; VIP = vasoactive intestinal polypeptide; CRF = corticotrophin-releasing factor. Reprinted from *American Journal of Surgery,* 182, Khelet H and Holte K, Review of postoperative ileus, 3S-10S, figure 6, Copyright © 2001, with permission from Excerpta Medica.

Intuitively, inflammation appears to be a reasonable culprit in the development of postoperative ileus and it would appear to be so, although not in the first twelve hours following surgery. Kalff et al. in 1998 demonstrated that manipulation of rat intestine resulted in an increase in the number of macrophages in the muscularis portion of the intestine as well as up-regulation of mast cells, T cells, and NK cells. Furthermore, the prevalence of inflammatory cells was related to the degree of surgical stimulation.[21] In a subsequent study it was shown that experimental smooth muscle dysfunction in rats may be attributable to the infiltration of inflammatory cells into the muscularis portion of the intestine.[22] The presence of this response in humans is assumed rather than defined, and the degree to which these cells contribute to the overall picture of postoperative ileus remains to be determined. However, the presence of proinflammatory mediators may expose the deeper levels of muscle to noxious lumenal contents, thus impairing contractility, and these mediators may be more likely to impair neuromuscular transmission in the intestine.[3]

The development of postoperative bowel dysfunction is unlikely to be caused by a solitary factor. Most likely it is a combination of the all of constituents previously outlined. The fact that thus far an antagonist of each system only partially attenuates the development of postoperative ileus further suggests a multifactorial mechanism.

CONTRIBUTION OF PERIOPERATIVE AND POSTOPERATIVE OPIOIDS

Opioids slow intestinal transit time by varied and complex means. The administration of opioids in the perioperative and postoperative periods prolong the duration and enhance the degree of ileus. Opioid receptors were discovered in the gastrointestinal tract in 1972, but their effects on gastrointestinal transit are not limited to agonism of peripheral receptors. Central effects play a role also. In the stomach, opioids decrease gastric motility and increase antral and duodenal tone, resulting in delayed gastric emptying.[23]

By a combination of spasmic activity and periods of atony, movement through the small intestine is slowed. Agonism of opioid receptors results in increased tone with periodic spasms. There follows an increase in the amplitude of nonpropulsive rhythm segmental contractions with a concurrent reduction in propulsive contractions.[23,24] These effects are not equal as the ileum is less sensitive to the effects of opiates than the ileum.

The most significant effects of opiates are on the large intestine. The administration of opioids reduces the activity of propulsive contractions and increases large intestine tone to the level of spasm; similar to the small intestine there is an increase in amplitude in the nonpropulsive wave. This slows passage of feces through the lumen, which results in excessive drying out and hardening of the lumenal contents, further slowing passage.[23,25]

ROLE OF GENERAL ANESTHESIA IN POSTOPERATIVE BOWEL DYSFUNCTION

The administration of anesthesia to patients presenting for surgery alters bowel motility. The nature and degree depend on the type and duration of anesthesia. Many agents have been implicated including nitrous oxide, inhalational agents, neostigmine, and induction agents.[25]

The effects of nitrous oxide on closed gas spaces have been well described and are well-known. Diffusion of this commonly used gas into the bowel lumen can distend the bowel; however, the effect on gastrointestinal motility is less certain. The use of nitrous oxide in gastrointestinal surgery has been shown to cause a delay in return of function and patients who received nitrous oxide, demonstrated by significantly longer hospital stays than those who received an air/oxygen mixture. Delay in return of bowel function may be the result of nitrous-oxide-induced distension, while secreted water and electrolytes worsen the extent and severity of gastrointestinal disturbances.[26]

Both halothane and enflurane have been shown not only to depress electromechanical activity in the bowel by both central and peripheral effects but also to reduce gastrointestinal contractility. However, these effects are transient and resolve 15 to 20 min after discontinuation of the agents.[25,27-30] There is insufficient published data regarding newer agents; however, whatever effect they may have would appear to be transitory and have minimal effect on more long-term ileus.

The effect of the commonly used intravenous induction agents such as thiopentone and propofol appears to be minimal.[30] Propofol has been shown to impair acetylcholine-mediated contraction at clinically relevant concentrations (serum propofol >1.2 µg/mL). But at higher concentrations (>4.8 µg/mL) spontaneous activity of both gastric and colonic smooth muscle is depressed.[31]

THERAPY OF POSTOPERATIVE BOWEL DYSFUNCTION

Nonpharmacological Therapies

Nasogastric Intubation

Since 1884 decompression of the stomach by the passage of a large bore nasogastric tube has been the mainstay of therapy for postoperative ileus.[32] There is no debate that "drip and suck" therapy improves the comfort of the patient; however, it has not been shown to affect the duration, or severity of postoperative ileus.[25] Investigators who compared patients having colonic resection with and without nasogastric intubation found no significant differences between the groups with respect to length of hospital stay, duration of ileus, gastric dilation, and operative complications.[33] The results of this study were repeated in another study of 97 patients, but in these groups the intubated (nasogastric) patients had significantly greater fluid loss. However, the volume of fluid administered was the same in both groups, and the authors suggested that the presence of a nasogastric tube might promote aerophagia and worsen abdominal distension already present.[25,34] Although adequate hydration and maintenance of electrolytes is essential postoperatively, nasogastric intubation should be reserved for individual patients, as need dictates, rather than routinely performed.[1]

Electrical Stimulation

Attempts have been made to emulate the success of cardiac pacing by using electrical stimulation to encourage gastrointestinal motility. Bilgutay et al. stimulated the stomach with the tip of a nasogastric tube in dogs and humans with paralytic ileus. Using fluoroscopy, they demonstrated an increase in gastric contractions and gastric emptying.[35] But a subsequent randomized controlled trial failed to show any benefit of this type of stimulation on gastrointestinal ileus.[36] The same level of success applies to the application of external magnetic energy.[37] The presence of smooth muscle hyperpolarization in postoperative ileus inhibits the development of spike potentials, making it unlikely that the application of an external current would overcome ileus.[8]

Early Enteral Nutrition

The presence of food in the gastrointestinal lumen stimulates the secretion of gastrointestinal hormones and commences the intestino-intestinal reflexes, which initiate coordinated propulsive activity. Most patients are fasted postoperatively for four to five days or until the return of bowel sounds, at which time they are commenced on a gradually evolving diet. The traditional wait for the return of bowel sounds not only encourages further catabolism and morbidity but may also be flawed as the absence of bowel sounds reflects the reaction of the bowel to fasting and does not necessarily predict its response to food. Early enteral nutrition has been the subject of a number of studies with variable outcomes. Several studies have found early enteral nutrition to be safe and to reduce the duration of postoperative ileus (Figure 7.2).[1,38-43] However, two more recent trials found no difference in duration of ileus or length of hospital stay.[44,45]

An important factor not accounted for was the type of analgesia used when assessing ileus and early enteral feeding. Postoperative ileus was reviewed by Holte and Kehlet who felt that if postoperative analgesia had not been managed with parenteral opiates, the result may have been more sympathetic to early feeding.[1] It would appear that there are benefits to early enteral feeding, which need to be elucidated further.

Preoperative Fiber Ingestion

Gastrointestinal motility has been shown to be influenced by dietary fiber, which reduces overall transit time by lowering intralumenal pressure and increasing the distension of intestinal walls. In a study of patients undergoing gynecological and obstetric procedures, the addition of bran to their preoperative diet led to a significant reduction in the duration of postoperative ileus compared with those who remained on their accustomed diet. These investigators felt

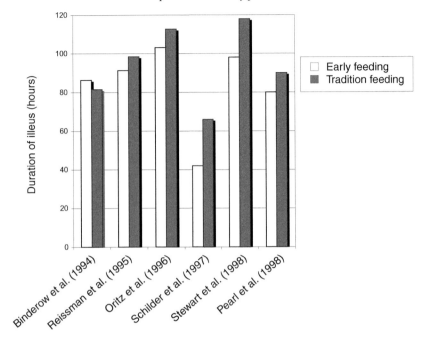

FIGURE 7.2. Randomized clinical trials assessing the effect of early enteral feeding versus traditional feeding on the resolution of ileus. *Source:* Holte K, Kehlet H. Postoperative ileus: A preventable event. *Br J Surg* 2000;87:1480-1493. © British Journal of Surgery Society Ltd. Reproduced with permission. Permission is granted by John Wiley & Sons Ltd. on behalf of the BJSS Ltd.

that incorporation of bran into a patient's diet should begin at least eight to ten days prior to surgery. Another study indicated that an eight-day treatment regimen of high fiber diet resulted in a faster resolution of postoperative ileus following elective cholecystectomy. The results of these two studies indicate that a simple intervention such as increased dietary fiber may speed the resolution of postoperative ileus.[46,47]

Perioperative Fluid Administration

When Gan et al. used a goal directed (cardiac output) protocol to estimate fluid requirements intraoperatively, the protocol patients received more fluid and had less postoperative complications than the control group.[48] Perioperative fluid administration was guided by cardiac output (esophageal doppler monitor) rather than traditional estimates of intraoperative dehydration (heart rate, urinary output, central venous pressure, systolic blood pressure). Patients in the protocol group received more hetastarch at 6 percent (843 mL versus 282 mL), had a shorter hospital stay (5 days versus 7 days), and experienced earlier toleration of oral solid regimen (3 days versus 4.7 days). Indeed, indexes of tissue hypoperfusion (gastric pH, arterial base excess) correlate with the development of postoperative complications, of which gastrointestinal disturbance was the most common in a study carried out by Bennett-Guerrero et al.[49] A number of studies have shown a direct relationship between hypovolemia and gut hypoperfusion (as indicated by gastric pH < 7.32);[50,51] thus, optimization of perioperative fluids may reduce the incidence of postoperative gastrointestinal dysfunction.

The converse of this is that excess fluid administration in the perioperative period may cause sufficient edema of the bowel wall to slow transit and so prolong the duration of postoperative ileus.[52] When postoperative patients were assigned to either a liberal fluid regimen (minimum of 3 L water and 154 mmol sodium per day) or a restrictive fluid regimen (maximum 2 L water and 77 mmol sodium per day), the length of postoperative ileus was significantly reduced in the restrictive group.[53,54] However, the overall morbidity associated with an inadequate and restrictive fluid regimen and the potential problems of gut hypoperfusion would suggest that perioperative fluid optimization is the most prudent course.

Surgical Technique

Studies have indicated that laparoscopic surgery results in earlier return of gastrointestinal function and earlier resolution of normal myoelectrical activity when compared with conventional open approaches. A number of controlled studies have shown earlier resolution of postoperative ileus when compared with open procedures (see Figure 7.3).[2] In three out of four studies there was a significant difference in the time to resolution of ileus between the open and laparoscopic groups.[55-58] The proposed mechanisms for this improvement include reduced activation of inhibitory reflexes and reduced inflam-

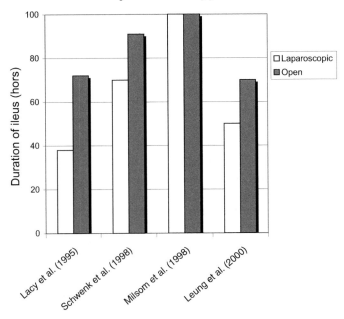

FIGURE 7.3. Randomized controlled clinical trials comparing the effect of open versus closed colonic surgery on ileus. *Source:* Reprinted from *American Journal of Surgery,* 182, Kehlet H, Holte K. Review of postoperative ileus, pp. 3S-10S, Copyright 2001, with permission from Exerpta Medica, Inc.

matory response locally. Most authors feel that more prospective controlled studies need to be performed to completely clarify this, but the trend toward minimally invasive surgery continues for a variety of other benefits.[1]

Psychological Preparation

Specific instructions given to patients preoperatively have been shown to shorten the duration of postoperative ileus.[59] Investigators randomized patients into one of two groups. Each group received a different five-minute presentation and was told that their adherence to these instructions would affect their recovery. The control group was given instructions unrelated to gastrointestinal motility and the experimental group was given specific instructions aimed at resolving ileus.

Both groups experienced ileus, but the experimental group's symptoms resolved earlier (2.6 days versus 4.1 days) and their duration of hospital stay was shorter by 1.5 days. The value of this technique in treating postoperative ileus may not be appreciated by all, but it does serve as a useful strategy.

Early Mobilization

Prolonged immobilization following surgery has never been shown to be of any benefit, but it does increase the risks of postoperative complications. However, when colonic motility was measured in healthy volunteers before, during, and after exercise, colonic motility was reduced as a result of exercise. Both the incidence of pressure waves and the area under the curve were significantly lower during exercise.[60] Waldhausen and Schirmer hypothesized that early ambulation following laparotomy would aid in restoration of normal gastrointestinal function. Unfortunately, the results of their study did not confirm this.[61] They positioned seromuscular myoelectric electrodes in the stomach, jejenum, and transverse colon of 35 patients at the time of laparotomy, ten of whom were exposed to an early ambulation regime. They concluded that ambulation had no overall effect on promoting an early recovery of normal gastrointestinal myoelectric activity. As early ambulation is beneficial in reducing the incidence of deep vein thrombosis and muscle atrophy, its use following surgery should continue and be encouraged.

Pharmacological Therapies

Agents Acting on Autonomic Nervous System

Normal gastrointestinal motility depends on balanced interaction between the parasympathetic and sympathetic nervous system. It has been suggested that a contributing factor to postoperative ileus is relative sympathetic overactivity and parasympathetic underactivity. Therefore, it would seem logical that inhibition of the sympathetic nervous system or agonism of the parasympathetic nervous system might improve postoperative ileus. Parasympathomimetic agents may be true cholinergic agonists or anticholinesterase inhibitors. True cholinergic agonists, which stimulate gastrointestinal function, possess muscarinic rather than nicotinic actions of acetylcholine and include agents such as bethanechol, carbachol, and methacholine. Studies performed in the 1970s examined the use of these agents in the treatment of postoperative ileus. Bethanechol, administered to humans, directly stimulated muscarinic receptors in the gut and improved ileus. Similar reports exist for carbachol in rat studies.[62,63] Continuing and more powerful data exists regarding the use of cholinesterase inhibitors for treating bowel dysfunction. A number of randomized studies have indicated that neostigmine given postoperatively is effective in increasing the magnitude and frequency of gastrointestinal pressure waves and in reducing the duration of ileus. However, its side effect profile necessitates intensive monitoring during administration and may, in fact, cause strong contractions.[25,64] Also, the administration of neostigmine is associated with an increased incidence of postoperative nausea and vomiting.[65]

Theoretically, an adrenergic blockade ought to affect the duration of postoperative ileus. However, most agents causing sympathetic blockade appear to have sufficient deleterious effects on the cardiovascular system as to limit their use in postoperative ileus. Whether an alpha, beta, or combined blockade is more effective is not clear. A number of studies have examined the benefits of administering propranolol to patients at risk of developing postoperative ileus. Some have had success, and no benefit has accrued in others. Hallerback and co-workers administered propranolol intravenously to patients undergoing bowel surgery and found a significantly shorter duration of postoperative ileus with no apparent adverse effects.[66] But when propranolol was administered orally to schistosomotic patients suffering postoperative ileus, no reduction in duration of POI or improvement in myoelectrical activity accrued.[67] A combination of neostigmine and propranolol (initially parenteral then oral) resulted in significant reduction in the duration of postoperative ileus when compared to neostigmine alone or placebo. No adverse effects were reported.[66] These studies were limited by sample size and manner of administration, but a larger well-controlled study on the effect of beta blockade is needed to clarify matters, particularly given the potential cardiac benefits of perioperative beta blockade.

Prokinetic Agents

Metoclopramide. Metoclopramide was introduced into clinical practice as antiemetic agent with both central and peripheral sites of activity. Its peripheral mode of action relies on its antidopaminergic activity, which results in the blockade of the normally inhibitory dopamine receptors in the gastrointestinal tract. The net effect of this is an increase in ion amplitude and frequency of gastric contractions, faster gastric emptying, and acceleration of transit time from duodenum to cecum, which should improve function in postoperative ileus. However, it has been studied many times and with many end points with the same conclusion. It does not reduce the duration or severity of postoperative ileus.[1,25,54] If metoclopramide had an innocuous side effect profile, its ineffectiveness might be excused, but the potential dystonic effect, drowsiness, and cardiac complications limit its potential usefulness. Henzi et al. analyzed 66 randomized, controlled studies examining the antiemetic efficacy of metoclopramide in 6,000 patients. They concluded that, in currently recommended doses, it is an ineffective antiemetic agent despite its use for almost 40 years.[68]

Cisapride. Cisapride, like metoclopramide, is a benzamide and a prokinetic. However, it does not appear to have any dopamine antagonist activity but rather increases the release of acetylcholine from postganglionic nerve endings in the myenteric plexus. This release of acetylcholine may be mediated by 5-hydroxytryptamine (5HT) or serotonin, as cisapride is an agonist of $5HT_4$ and an antagonist of $5HT_3$ receptors.[69,70] As a prokinetic, cisapride affects the whole gastrointestinal tract. Gastric emptying is accelerated,[71] both small bowel and colonic motor activity are increased, and the transit time from ileum to rectum is reduced.[72] The effectiveness of cisapride as a therapy for postoperative ileus has been studied a number of times in prospective randomized trials with varied results. In two studies where cisapride was administered intravenously, there was reduction in time to remission of ileus, although at least two administrations were required.[73,74] However, in another study when cisapride was administered rectally there was no reduction in time to passage of stool.[75] Whatever the benefits of cisapride in the treatment of postoperative ileus the prevalence of cardiac adverse effects is cause for concern. As $5HT_4$ receptors are present not only in the gastrointestinal tract but also the urinary tract and the cardiovascular system, cisapride has been reported to be responsible for urinary incontinence and supraventricular tachycardia. The most sinister effects appear to be related to cisapride's class III antiarrythmic effects. This may result in predisposed individuals, in prolongation of the QT interval and torsades de pointes.[76-78]

Erythromycin. The enterocromaffin cells of the proximal small intestine secrete a peptide hormone, motilin, which stimulates the MMC and increases motility. The administration of the macrolide antibiotic erythromycin may result in abdominal cramping which is caused by agonism of motilin receptors.[25] Erythromycin has been shown to reduce gastric emptying time in diabetic gastroparesis but has not been shown to improve the duration or severity of postoperative ileus. This appears to be, in part, due to the fact that there is a gradual reduction in the concentration of motilin receptors along the gastrointestinal tract, with the highest concentrations in the gastric antrum and proximal duodenum.[79,80]

Prostaglandins

The presence and activity of prostaglandins throughout the gastrointestinal tract has long been established.[25] In 1980 Ruwart and coworkers published a study in which they demonstrated the positive effects of prostaglandin E_2 and 16-16 dimethyl prostaglandin E_2 on gastric, small intestinal, and colonic motility in laparotomized rats.[81] The effects of prostaglandins are exerted at both a muscular and neural level. Mulholland and Simeone demonstrated that prostaglandin E_2 increased acetylcholine release from myenteric plexus neurons.[82] However, the benefits of parenteral or oral prostaglandins on postoperative ileus in humans remains to be proven. Yokoyama et al. indicated that PG-$F_{2\alpha}$ was not as effective in resolving ileus as Leu-13 motilin.[83] The importance of prostaglandins in the therapy of postoperative ileus becomes more significant when they are inhibited by cyclooxygenase inhibitors.

Laxatives

Despite the widespread use of laxatives in the treatment of bowel dysfunction, there is little evidence of their benefit in postoperative ileus. The only published study on the effects of postoperative laxatives in ileus was nonrandomized with no control group.[84] Milk of

magnesia and biscolic suppositories were administered to 20 conse-
cutives patients following radical hysterectomy. Return of flatus occurred at three days and discharge at four days, which compared
favorably with a previous study by these authors; however, a blinded,
randomized, controlled trial would be beneficial to show a statistically significant difference.

Cholecystokinin

Cholecystokinin (CCK) is a peptide hormone produced by gastrointestinal mucosa whose major function is to stimulate gallbladder
contraction and pancreatic secretion.[85] It has been shown to have
prokinetic effects; however, it has not been shown to affect the duration of postoperative ileus in randomized studies.[54] Ceruletide, a
CCK agonist, has been shown to reduce the duration of ileus in two
studies.[86,87] But the benefits are limited, due to the propensity of
ceruletide to cause nausea and vomiting and thus requiring additional
antiemetic therapy.

Opioid Antagonists

Postoperative bowel dysfunction and ileus have many contributing
factors, which have been discussed. The antagonism of the gastrointestinal effects of opiates would seem a rational way of reducing the
duration and severity of postoperative ileus. The peripherally positioned opiate receptors appear to be the predominant receptors in mediating postoperative bowel dysfunction. The problem, however, is
that postoperative opiates serve an important purpose in reducing
postoperative pain and traditional antagonists inhibit the peripheral
and central effects of opiates. The challenge is to maximize analgesia
without compromising gastrointestinal function—that is, antagonize
peripheral gastrointestinal effects of opiates without affecting central
analgesic mechanisms.

Naloxone. Selective antagonism of the μ opiate receptor is
achieved easily by administration of naloxone. However, naloxone
readily crosses the blood-brain barrier and therefore even low doses
easily reverse analgesia. Oral naloxone has 2 percent bioavailability
due to first-pass metabolism and orally is effective in restoring and
improving gastrointestinal function if impaired by opiate use. Despite this, there is a gradual dose-dependent increase in plasma con-

centrations of unmetabolized and active naloxone, which can reduce analgesia prior to effective improvement in gastrointestinal function.[88] For this reason naloxone remains an unviable treatment of postoperative ileus in patients.

Methylnaltrexone. The aim in achieving remission or prevention of opioid-induced bowel dysfunction is to develop compounds which are selective antagonists of the peripheral opiate receptors. The development of a quaternary derivative of the μ receptor antagonist naltrexone has created a μ receptor antagonist that is poorly lipid soluble, does not penetrate the central nervous system, and thus does not antagonize the central analgesic effects of opiates or precipitate withdrawal.[89-91] Methylnaltrexone (MNTX) exhibits a lack of central activity in animal models. When MNTX was administered to opioid-tolerant dogs, no withdrawal response was elicited, despite withdrawal occurring on administration of 100-fold lower doses of naloxone.[90] MNTX, on subcutaneous administration, failed to reverse morphine-induced catalepsy in rats despite a 10,000-fold lower dose succeeding when administered intracerebrally.[89] It appears that MNTX is relatively resistant to the effects of demethylation, which plague other quaternary antagonist derivatives, such as methylnaloxone, and thus is more peripherally selective.[90,91] Its direct gastrointestinal effects have been demonstrated on guinea pig ileum and human small intestine muscle strips when MNTX reversed morphine-induced inhibition of electrically stimulated contractions.[91] Yuan and co-workers administered MNTX to healthy human volunteers who were also given morphine. Oral MNTX prevented the morphine- induced delay in orocecal transit time and preserved analgesia.[92] In a later study, administration of enteric-coated MNTX orally was six times more efficient at preventing morphine-induced transit time than an uncoated version.[93] The enteric coating, prevented gastric absorption, was associated with less plasma bioavailability than uncoated, but had greater efficacy than the uncoated version, further reinforcing the direct lumenal activity of the agent.

As yet there are no published reports of MNTX effects on postoperative ileus. MNTX remains an interesting and potentially very useful drug in this arena.[94]

Alvimopan (ADL 8-2698). Alvimopan is a new μ receptor antagonist that has recently undergone Phase III trials. Its large molecular weight, zwitterionic structure, and polarity prevent it from being readily absorbed by the gastrointestinal tract or from crossing the blood-brain barrier. These properties make it an ideal agent for treating opioid-induced bowel dysfunction, and many studies have examined its efficacy in this regard.

As has been discussed, the impact of opioids on bowel dysfunction and postoperative ileus is due primarily to μ receptor agonism, so it would seem wise that alvimopan binds with more affinity to this receptor than to κ or δ, which is what it does. It has no inherent agonist activity, nor does it have any affinity for adrenergic, dopaminergic, or GABA receptors.[94] Early animal investigation demonstrated its ability to relieve opioid-induced gastrointestinal dysfunction without precipitating withdrawal.[95] The ability of alvimopan to relieve opiate-induced constipation in human subjects was examined by Barr and co-workers. When administered with morphine and compared with placebo, alvimopan was associated with faster gastrointestinal transit, increased stool number, and increased stool weight.[96]

In contrast with MNTX, the effects of alvimopan on postoperative ileus have been examined. Taguchi and fellow investigators examined the effects of orally administered alvimopan on patients scheduled for either partial colectomy or hysterectomy who received either morphine or meperidine for analgesia.[97] Patients received either alvimopan 1mg, alvimopan 6 mg, or placebo two hours before surgery and twice daily after surgery until the first bowel movement. The time to first bowel movement was significantly shorter in the group that received 6 mg compared to the other two groups. This group was also discharged one day earlier and had less postoperative nausea and vomiting than the other two groups. Of all the agents suggested for the treatment of postoperative bowel dysfunction influenced by opiates, alvimopan seems the most promising. Therapeutic options for postoperative ileus are summarized in Table 7.2.

Alternatives, Adjuncts, and Benefits

Epidural Analgesia

If opioids administered parenterally add to the gastrointestinal dysfunction already present due to the trauma and manipulation of surgery, logic would suggest that complete or partial avoidance of these contributory agents should influence outcome. Minimizing opioids and achieving adequate postoperative pain control remains a

TABLE 7.2. Therapeutic options for postoperative ileus.

Nonpharmacological	Pharmacological
Nasogastric intubation	Agents acting on autonomic nervous system
Electrical stimulation	Prokinetic agents
Early enteral nutrition	Metoclopramide
Preoperative fiber	Cisparide
Perioperative fluids	Erythromycin
Surgical technique	Prostaglandins
Psychological preparation	Laxatives
Early mobilization	Cholecystokinin
	Opiate antagonists
	Naloxone
	Methylnaltrexone
	Alvimopan

very high priority for surgeons and anesthesiologists alike. Using epidurally administered local anesthetics and narcotics is a tried and accepted method of attaining this. Not only does postoperative epidural blockade achieve analgesia and reduce dependence on opiate analgesia, the blockade of thoracolumbar sympathetic fibers while leaving the craniosacral parasympathetic input intact would be expected to leave gastrointestinal motility intact.[98] Systemic infusions of lidocaine have been shown to increase gastrointestinal motility in postoperative ileus.[99] The theoretical beneficial effects of epidural anesthesia are as follows:

- Blockade of nociceptive afferent nerves
- Blockade of thoracolumbar sympathetic efferent nerves
- Unopposed parasympathetic efferent nerves
- Reduced need for postoperative opiates
- Increased gastrointestinal blood flow
- Systemic absorption of local anesthetic[98]

Numerous studies have examined the effects of epidural infusion on postoperative ileus with mixed results, as is illustrated in Figure 7.4.[98] In all studies examined, the duration of ileus was shorter in those who received epidural anesthesia, but in some the duration was not statistically significant.[100-109] Statistical significance is achieved in studies where the catheter is placed above T12, where there appears to be less benefit when a lumbar epidural is placed for abdomi-

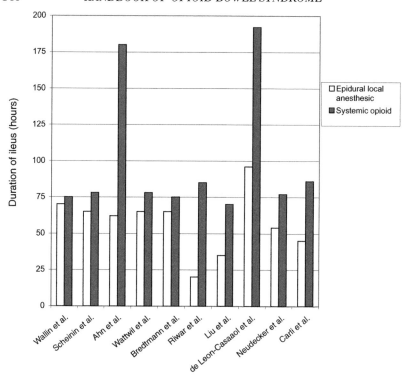

FIGURE 7.4. Randomized clinical trials assessing the effects of epidural local anesthetics versus systemic opioids on postoperative ileus. *Source:* Holte K, Kehlet H. Postoperative ileus: A preventable event. *Br J Surg* 2000;87:1480-1493. © British Journal of Surgery Society Ltd. Reproduced with permission. Permission is granted by John Wiley & Sons Ltd. on behalf of the BJSS Ltd.

nal surgery.[98] In no case has systemic analgesia been associated with more rapid recovery of gastrointestinal motility. Scott and co-workers compared thoracic epidural analgesia, lumbar epidural analgesia, and intravenous PCA (patient controlled analgesia)-administered morphine.[110] Bowel sounds returned significantly earlier in the thoracic group (2.45 ± 1.19 days) when compared with the lumbar epidural group (3.17 ± 1.18 days) and the PCA group (2.96 ± 1.14 days). A similar significant difference applied to timing of first bowel movement. In a review of the effects of epidural analgesia on gastrointestinal motility, Steinbrook identified seven studies in which the effects on postoperative ileus of thoracic epidurals administering either local anesthetics or opioids were examined.[98] In all seven studies, gastrointestinal motility was greater with the use of epidural local anesthetics compared with epidural narcotics. Liu et al. compared the use of epidural bupivacaine and morphine, epidural morphine alone, and epidural bupivacaine alone.[106] They found the shortest duration of ileus in the groups that received epidural bupivacaine (40 ± 2 hours) and epidural morphine/bupivacaine (43 ± 4 hours), compared with epidural morphine alone (71 ± 4 hours) or PCA morphine (81 ± 3 hours).

Overall, there are many benefits to postoperative epidural analgesia, and their effects on postoperative bowel function cannot be ignored. However, to be of maximum benefit, the epidural must be inserted above T12, and local anesthetics should be administered via catheter either alone or with an opiate.

Tramadol

Tramadol is a synthetic 4-phenylpiperidine analog of codeine (see Figure 7.5).[111] It is a centrally acting analgesic agent with two modes of action: It is a weak μ receptor agonist (6,000-fold less than morphine) with some affinity for δ and κ receptors, and it inhibits the reuptake of serotonin and norepinephrine. Although the nonopioid mechanism of action would appear to be the dominant (in view of the weak affinity for the opiate receptor), the two systems appear to work synergistically.[112]

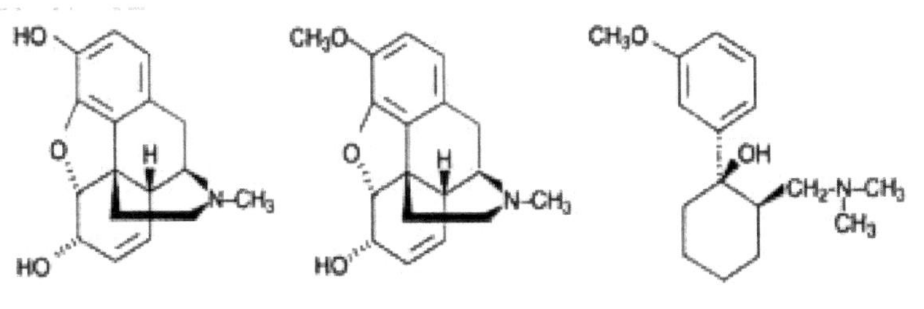

FIGURE 7.5. Chemical structures of morphine (left), codeine (center), and tramadol (right). *Source:* Originally published in Lewis KS, Han NH. Tramadol: A new centrally acting analgesic. *Am J Health Syst Pharm* 1997;54:643-652. © 1997, American Society of Health-System Pharmacists, Inc. All rights reserved. Reprinted with permission. (R0509).

The perioperative use of tramadol has been assessed in several randomized double-blind parallel group studies. Tramadol has been shown to effectively relieve moderate to severe pain associated with several types of surgery (including abdominal, orthopedic, and cardiac). Tramadol administered via PCA has been examined on a number of occasions and found to effectively treat moderate to severe pain. In five studies where tramadol was compared with opioids (morphine, oxycodone), it was found to be at least as effective as the opioids studied.[112] Although tramadol does have some μ receptor activity, its weak agonism appears to have little effect on gastrointestinal motility.

The effects of tramadol on gastrointestinal function have been investigated in healthy volunteers in a number of randomized, controlled studies. Crighton et al. assessed the comparative effects of morphine, codeine, and tramadol on gastric emptying in healthy volunteers using the paracetemol (acetaminophen) absorption test. They concluded that although morphine profoundly inhibited gastric emptying, tramadol measurably slowed gastric emptying but this did not reach statistical significance.[113] Another small study contradicted this when gastric emptying was assessed by applied potential tomography; however, this was not compared with the effects of morphine.[114] Wilder-Smith and colleagues in 1999 assessed the effects of tramadol on somatic and visceral sensation and gastrointestinal function in 50 patients who had received postoperative infusions of morphine or tramadol.[115] They found that while pain was adequately and similarly well controlled with both techniques, gastrointestinal function returned one day earlier in the tramadol group.

As yet there are no published studies of the effects of tramadol on postoperative ileus, but if it is as effective an analgesic as the available evidence suggests, its poor opiate receptor agonist properties may mean it is an effective agent for postoperative pain without affecting gastrointestinal function.

Nonsteroidal Anti-Inflammatory Drugs

Prostaglandins E_2 and I_2 mediate pain by lowering the threshold for stimulation of afferent nerve fibers by noxious stimuli such as histamine and bradykinin.[116-117] Nonsteroidal anti-inflammatory drugs (NSAIDs) inhibit the cyclooxygenase enzyme and, therefore, inhibit the synthesis of prostaglandins. Furness and Costa in 1974 demonstrated that stimulation of these pain fibers leads to inhibition of small intestinal motility through reflex adrenergic pathways.[6]

If the production of prostaglandin is sufficiently high to exert a hyperalgesic effect, then the administration of NSAIDs in adequate quantities should improve ileus via their analgesic effects. Intraperitoneal ascetic acid creates a chemically induced paralytic ileus, which is mediated via this hyperalgesic route. In rats the expected reduction in gastrointestinal motility is prevented following pretreatment with NSAIDs (indomethacin, ketoprofen, piroxicam, and ximoprofen).[118] This occurred at analgesic doses, suggesting that in this model the effects are mediated via the analgesic properties of NSAIDs.

A second potential mechanism by which NSAIDs may affect gastrointestinal motility is through increased smooth muscle activity due to a reduction in the levels of inhibitory prostaglandins. Different prostaglandins exert different effects on the small intestinal motility. PgI_2 and PgE_2 inhibit motility, whereas $PgF_{2\alpha}$ and Pg_{D2} stimulate motility.[119] Kelley et al. studied the effects of ketorolac on a rat model of postoperative ileus. They found that, when administered preoperatively, ketorolac completely reversed the delay in gastrointestinal transit and inhibition of myoelectrical activity seen in postoperative ileus.[120] They postulated that the primary reason for this was the inhibition of all prostaglandin synthesis resulting in dominant inhibitory effects being reversed. In a later study, administration of salsalate improved postoperative bowel transit in rats, but the effect was lost by the concomitant administration of morphine.[121] NSAIDs exert their effects in many ways, but one of their primary benefits may be the reduction in opiate requirements in the postoperative period.

COX-2 Inhibitors

The initial step in prostaglandin synthesis is catalyzed by the cyclooxygenase (COX) enzyme. Two isoenzymes have been identified, COX-1 and COX-2. COX-1 is produced throughout the body and is essential to the formation of prostaglandins associated with platelet aggregation, gastrointestinal protection, and normal renal function. COX-2 is produced by inflammatory cells and catalyzes the production of prostaglandins associated with pathophysiological processes such as pain, inflammation, and fever.[122] The discovery of these two processes led to the development of inhibitors of cyclo-oxygenase-2 such as celecoxib, rofecoxib, valdecoxib, and its pro-drug parecoxib, to attain analgesic efficacy while minimizing NSAID side effects.

Many studies have examined the analgesic effects of COX-2 inhibitors, the majority of which have related to the treatment of painful musculoskeletal conditions such as rheumatoid arthritis and osteoarthritis. Similarly, the majority of studies of the effects of COX-2 inhibitors on acute postoperative pain have focused on orthopedic and dental procedures (see Table 7.3).

Gimbel et al. studied the efficacy of celecoxib versus a hydrocodone/acetaminophen combination for the treatment of postoperative orthopedic pain. They found that during the five-day postoperative study period patients who received celecoxib 200 mg t.i.d. had superior analgesia and tolerability compared to those who received hydrocodone 10 mg/acetaminophen 1,000 mg t.i.d.[123]

In a study carried out by Issioui et al., celecoxib 200 mg, rofexicib 50 mg, and ibuprofen 800 mg were compared with placebo for treatment of pain following ear, nose, and throat surgery.[124] All the drugs

TABLE 7.3. Indications and dosage recommendations for cyclooxygenase-2 inhibitors.

Drug	Indication	Dosage
Celecoxib	Osteoarthritis	200 mg QD or 100 mg BID
	Rheumatoid arthritis	100-200 mg BID
	Familial adenomatous polyposis	400 mg BID
	Acute pain and primary dysmenorrhea	400 mg initially, then 200 mg if needed then 200 mg BID PRN
Rofecoxib	Osteoarthritis	12.5-25 mg QD
	Rheumatoid arthritis	25 mg QD
	Acute pain	50 mg QD
	Primary dysmenorrhea	50 mg QD
Valdecoxib	Osteoarthritis	10 mg QD
	Rheumatoid arthritis	10 mg QD
	Primary dysmenorrhea	20 mg BID PRN

Source: Gajraj NM. Cyclooxygenase-2 inhibitors. *Anesth Analg* 2003;96:1720-1738. Reprinted with permission.

examined were found to be equipotent, and premedication with these agents reduced the need for postoperative analgesia. The only recently published study of the efficacy of COX-2 inhibition, following lower abdominal surgery, was carried out by Shen and Sinatra. They found that patients who received rofecoxib 50 mg one hour prior to surgery required 44 percent less morphine during the first twenty-four-hour period, had less pain on effort, and had better pulmonary function 12 hours after surgery, compared to placebo.[125] The fact that as analgesics such as COX-2 inhibitors reduce opiate requirements following surgery, while minimizing gastric and hemostatic side effects, would be enough to recommend them as agents that may minimize postoperative ileus. However, studies on rats have shown that there is an increase in cyclooxygenase-2 in rats who suffered postoperative ileus following intestinal manipulation, which led to an in vitro decrease in jejenal muscle activity and gastrointestinal transit.[126] The potential beneficial effects COX-2 inhibitors are summarized in Table 7.4.[127]

Others

The administration of alternative analgesic agents such as ketamine, while not per se affecting gastrointestinal function, reduces requirements for postoperative opiates.[128] Other agents, which have analgesic efficacy, such as clonidine and dexmedetomidine, may prove to be powerful adjuncts in minimizing the negative gastrointestinal effects of opiates.

TABLE 7.4. Use of COX-2 inhibitors perioperatively.

Advantages	Disadvantages
Opioid-sparing effect:	Similar renal risks to NSAIDs
Less ileus	Idiosyncratic GI problems
Less somnolence	Bone-healing issues in fractures
Less respiratory depression	Thromboembolic risk in susceptible patients
Less nausea/vomiting	
Less postoperative bleeding	
Reduced risk of gastrointestinal irritation	

Source: Ruoff G, Lema M. Strategies in pain management: New and potential indications for COX-2 specific inhibitors. *J Pain Symptom Manage* 2003;25: S21-S31.

CONCLUSIONS

The combination of intra-abdominal trauma, anesthesia, and analgesia make some degree of bowel dysfunction following surgery almost inevitable. There is no single cause and therefore no single cure; indeed, there are a number of causes. Thus, if postoperative bowel dysfunction is dealt with via a multimodal approach, its effects may be minimized. Good patient care, early enteral feeding, and adequate fluid resuscitation all have a role to play. The ever-decreasing level of surgical invasiveness reduces the amount of bowel manipulation and the degree of dysfunction that is experienced afterward. The effects of opioids can be and are minimized by using alternative analgesic techniques and agents such as nonsteroidal anti-inflammatory agents, tramadol, and regional and neuraxial anesthesia. The recent advent of drugs such as methylnaltrexone and alvimopan (see Chapters 10 and 11 of this book) suggest that the analgesic benefit of opioids can be great while their gastrointestinal side effects are minimal. Specific agents to treat established postoperative ileus are either ineffective or limited by side effects. However, further study of the mechanisms leading to ileus should shed some light on potential therapies, such as treatment aimed at the autonomic nervous system.

NOTES

1. Holte K, Kehlet H. Postoperative ileus: A preventable event. *Br J Surg* 2000;87:1480-1493.

2. Kehlet H, Holte K. Review of postoperative ileus. *Am J Surg* 2001;182: 3S-10S.

3. Prasad M, Matthews JB. Deflating postoperative ileus. *Gastroenterology* 1999;117:489-492.

4. Moss G, Regal ME, Lichtig L. Reducing postoperative pain, narcotics, and length of hospitalization. *Surgery* 1986;99:206-210.

5. Szurszewski JH. A migrating electric complex of canine small intestine. *Am J Physiol* 1969;217:1757-1763.

6. Luckey A, Livingston E, Tache Y. Mechanisms and treatment of postoperative ileus. *Arch Surg* 2003;138:206-214.

7. De Winter BY, Boeckxstaens GE, De Man JG, Moreels TG, Herman AG, Pelckmans PA. Effect of adrenergic and nitrergic blockade on experimental ileus in rats. *Br J Pharmacol* 1997;120:464-468.

8. Livingston EH, Passaro EP Jr. Postoperative ileus. *Digest Dis Sci* 1990; 35:121-132.

9. Dubois A, Kopin IJ, Pettigrew KD, Jacobowitz DM. Chemical and histochemical studies of postoperative sympathetic activity in the digestive tract in rats. *Gastroenterology* 1974;66:403-407.

10. Deloof S, Croix D, Tramu G. The role of vasoactive intestinal polypeptide in the inhibition of antral and pyloric electrical activity in rabbits. *J Auton Nerv Syst* 1988;22:167-173.

11. Holzer P, Lippe IT, Holzer-Petsche U. Inhibition of gastrointestinal transit due to surgical trauma or peritoneal irritation is reduced in capsaicin-treated rats. *Gastroenterology* 1986;91:360-363.

12. Kalff JC, Schraut WH, Billiar TR, Simmons RL, Bauer AJ. Role of inducible nitric oxide synthase in postoperative intestinal smooth muscle dysfunction in rodents. *Gastroenterology* 2000;118:316-327.

13. Freeman M, Cheng G, Hocking MP. Role of alpha- and beta-calcitonin gene-related peptide in postoperative small bowel ileus. *J Gastrointest Surg* 1999;3: 39-43.

14. Zittel TT, Reddy SN, Plourde V, Raybould HE. Role of spinal afferents and calcitonin gene-related peptide in the postoperative gastric ileus in anesthetized rats. *Ann Surg* 1994;219:79-87.

15. Terawaki Y, Takayanagi I, Takagi K. Effects of 5-hydroxytryptamine and morphine on the stomach motility in situ. *Jpn J Pharmacol* 1976:7-12.

16. Howd RA, Adamovics A, Palekar A. Naloxone and intestinal motility. *Experientia* 1978;34:1310-1311.

17. Konturek SJ, Thor P, Krol R, Dembinski A, Schally AV. Influence of methionine-enkephalin and morphine on myoelectric activity of small bowel. *Am J Physiol* 1980;238:G384-G389.

18. Barquist E, Zinner M, Rivier J, Tache Y. Abdominal surgery-induced delayed gastric emptying in rats: Role of CRF and sensory neurons. *Am J Physiol* 1992;262:G616-G620.

19. Tache Y, Monnikes H, Bonaz B, Rivier J. Role of CRF in stress-related alterations of gastric and colonic motor function. *Ann N Y Acad Sci* 1993;697:233-243.

20. Nozu T, Martinez V, Rivier J, Tache Y. Peripheral urocortin delays gastric emptying: Role of CRF receptor 2. *Am J Physiol* 1999;276:G867-G874.

21. Kalff JC, Schraut WH, Simmons RL, Bauer AJ. Surgical manipulation of the gut elicits an intestinal muscularis inflammatory response resulting in postsurgical ileus. *Ann Surg* 1998;228:652-663.

22. Kalff JC, Carlos TM, Schraut WH, Billiar TR, Simmons RL, Bauer AJ. Surgically induced leukocytic infiltrates within the rat intestinal muscularis mediate postoperative ileus. *Gastroenterology* 1999;117:378-387.

23. Reisine T, Posternak G. Opioid analgesics and antagonists. In Hardman JGG, Gilman A, Limbird LL (eds.), *Goodman & Gilman's The pharmacologic basis of therapeutics*. New York: McGraw-Hill; 1996.

24. Borody TJ, Quigley EM, Phillips SF, Wienbeck M, Tucker RL, Haddad A, Zinsmeister AR. Effects of morphine and atropine on motility and transit in the human ileum. *Gastroenterology* 1985;89:562-570.

25. Resnick J, Greenwald DA, Brandt LJ. Delayed gastric emptying and postoperative ileus after nongastric abdominal surgery: Part I. *Am J Gastroenterol* 1997;92:751-762.

26. Scheinin B, Lindgren L, Scheinin TM. Peroperative nitrous oxide delays bowel function after colonic surgery. *Br J Anaesth* 1990;64:154-158.

27. Marshall FN, Pittinger CB, Long JP. Effects of halothane on gastrointestinal motility. *Anesthesiology* 1961;22:363-366.

28. Schurizek BA, Willacy LH, Kraglund K, Andreasen F, Juhl B. Effects of general anaesthesia with enflurane on antroduodenal motility, pH and gastric emptying rate in man. *Eur J Anaesthesiol* 1989;6:265-279.

29. Schurizek BA, Willacy LH, Kraglund K, Andreasen F, Juhl B. Effects of general anaesthesia with halothane on antroduodenal motility, pH and gastric emptying rate in man. *Br J Anaesth* 1989;62:129-137.

30. Ogilvy AJ, Smith G. The gastrointestinal tract after anaesthesia. *Eur J Anaesthesiol Suppl* 1995;10:35-42.

31. Lee TL, Ang SB, Dambisya YM, Adaikan GP, Lau LC. The effect of propofol on human gastric and colonic muscle contractions. *Anesth Analg* 1999; 89:1246-1249.

32. Kussmaul C. Heilung von ileus durch magenausspulung. *Berl Klin Wochenschr* 1984;21:669-685.

33. Colvin DB, Lee W, Eisenstat TE, Rubin RJ, Salvati EP. The role of nasointestinal intubation in elective colonic surgery. *Dis Colon Rectum* 1986; 29:295-299.

34. Reasbeck PG, Rice ML, Herbison GP. Nasogastric intubation after intestinal resection. *Surgery, Gynecology & Obstetrics* 1984;158:354-358.

35. Bilgutay AM, Wingrove R, Griffen WO, Bonnabeau RC, Jr., Lillehei CW. Gastro-intestinal pacing: A new concept in the treatment of ileus. *Ann Surg* 1963; 158:338-348.

36. Berger T, Kewenter J, Kock NG. Response to gastrointestinal pacing: Antral, duodenal and jejunal motility in control and postoperative patients. *Ann Surg* 1966;164:139-144.

37. Barker P, Allcutt D, McCollum CN. Pulsed electromagnetic energy fails to prevent postoperative ileus. *J R Coll Surg Edinb* 1984;29:147-150.

38. Binderow SR, Cohen SM, Wexner SD, Nogueras JJ. Must early postoperative oral intake be limited to laparoscopy? *Dis Colon Rectum* 1994;37:584-589.

39. Reissman P, Teoh TA, Cohen SM, Weiss EG, Nogueras JJ, Wexner SD. Is early oral feeding safe after elective colorectal surgery? A prospective randomized trial. *Ann Surg* 1995;222:73-77.

40. Ortiz H, Armendariz P, Yarnoz C. Is early postoperative feeding feasible in elective colon and rectal surgery?[comment]. *International Journal of Colorectal Disease* 1996;11:119-121.

41. Schilder JM, Hurteau JA, Look KY, Moore DH, Raff G, Stehman FB, Sutton GP. A prospective controlled trial of early postoperative oral intake following major abdominal gynecologic surgery. *Gynecol Oncol* 1997;67:235-240.

42. Pearl ML, Valea FA, Fischer M, Mahler L, Chalas E. A randomized controlled trial of early postoperative feeding in gynecologic oncology patients undergoing intra-abdominal surgery. *Obstet Gynecol* 1998;92:94-97.

43. Stewart BT, Woods RJ, Collopy BT, Fink RJ, Mackay JR, Keck JO. Early feeding after elective open colorectal resections: A prospective randomized trial. *Aust NZ J Surg* 1998;68:125-128.

44. Heslin MJ, Latkany L, Leung D, Brooks AD, Hochwald SN, Pisters PW, Shike M, Brennan MF. A prospective, randomized trial of early enteral feeding after resection of upper gastrointestinal malignancy. *Ann Surg* 1997;226:567-577; discussion 577-580.

45. Watters JM, Kirkpatrick SM, Norris SB, Shamji FM, Wells GA. Immediate postoperative enteral feeding results in impaired respiratory mechanics and decreased mobility. *Ann Surg* 1997;226:369-77; discussion 377-380.

46. Sculati O, Bard M, Ficher D, Radrizzani D, Paganoni A, Giampiccoli A, Lanzetta V, Lapichino G, Manenti G. A simple method for resolving postoperative ileus in an early stage in obstetric and gynecological surgery. *Curr Ther Reasch-Clinical Exp* 1981;29:997-1002.

47. Sculati O, Giampiccoli G, Gozzi B, Minissale V, Zambetti N, Iapichino G, Ipezzoli C, Giacomelli M, Lazzari P, Franzosi MG. Bran diet for an earlier resolution of post-operative ileus. *J Int Med Res* 1982;10:194-197.

48. Gan TJ, Soppitt A, Maroof M, el-Moalem H, Robertson KM, Moretti E, Dwane P, Glass PS. Goal-directed intraoperative fluid administration reduces length of hospital stay after major surgery. *Anesthesiology* 2002;97:820-826.

49. Bennett-Guerrero E, Welsby I, Dunn TJ, Young LR, Wahl TA, Diers TL, Phillips-Bute BG, Newman MF, Mythen MG. The use of a postoperative morbidity survey to evaluate patients with prolonged hospitalization after routine, moderate-risk, elective surgery. *Anesth Analg* 1999;89:514-519.

50. Mythen MG, Webb AR. Intra-operative gut mucosal hypoperfusion is associated with increased post-operative complications and cost. *Intensive Care Med* 1994;20:99-104.

51. Mythen MG, Webb AR. Perioperative plasma volume expansion reduces the incidence of gut mucosal hypoperfusion during cardiac surgery. *Arch Surg* 1995;130:423-429.

52. Holte K, Sharrock NE, Kehlet H. Pathophysiology and clinical implications of perioperative fluid excess. *Br J Anaesth* 2002;89:622-632.

53. Lobo DN, Bostock KA, Neal KR, Perkins AC, Rowlands BJ, Allison SP. Effect of salt and water balance on recovery of gastrointestinal function after elective colonic resection: A randomised controlled trial. *Lancet* 2002;359:1812-1818.

54. Holte K, Kehlet H. Postoperative ileus: Progress toward effective management. *Drugs* 2002;62:2603-2615.

55. Lacy AM, Garcia-Valdecasas JC, Pique JM, Delgado S, Campo E, Bordas JM, Taura P, Grande L, Fuster J, Pacheco JL. Short-term outcome analysis of a randomized study comparing laparoscopic vs open colectomy for colon cancer. *Surg Endosc* 1995;9:1101-1105.

56. Milsom JW, Bohm B, Hammerhofer KA, Fazio V, Steiger E, Elson P. A prospective, randomized trial comparing laparoscopic versus conventional techniques in colorectal cancer surgery: a preliminary report. *J Am Coll Surg* 1998;187:46-54; discussion 54-55.

57. Schwenk W, Bohm B, Haase O, Junghans T, Muller JM. Laparoscopic versus conventional colorectal resection: A prospective randomised study of postoperative ileus and early postoperative feeding. *Langenbecks Arch Surg* 1998;383:49-55.

58. Leung KL, Lai PB, Ho RL, Meng WC, Yiu RY, Lee JF, Lau WY. Systemic cytokine response after laparoscopic-assisted resection of rectosigmoid carcinoma: A prospective randomized trial. *Ann Surg* 2000;231:506-511.

59. Disbrow EA, Bennett HL, Owings JT. Effect of preoperative suggestion on postoperative gastrointestinal motility. *West J Med* 1993;158:488-492.

60. Rao SS, Beaty J, Chamberlain M, Lambert PG, Gisolfi C. Effects of acute graded exercise on human colonic motility. *Am J Physiol* 1999;276:G1221-G1226.

61. Waldhausen JH, Schirmer BD. The effect of ambulation on recovery from postoperative ileus. *Ann Surg* 1990;212:671-677.

62. Ruwart MJ, Klepper MS, Rush BD. Carbachol stimulation of gastrointestinal transit in the postoperative Ileus rat. *J Surg Res* 1979;26:18-26.

63. Furness JB, Costa M. Adynamic ileus, its pathogenesis and treatment. *Med Biol* 1974;52:82-89.

64. Herschman Z. Other ways to stimulate postoperative bowel function. *Anesth Analg* 1998;87:500.

65. King MJ, Milazkiewicz R, Carli F, Deacock AR. Influence of neostigmine on postoperative vomiting. *Br J Anaesth* 1988;61:403-406.

66. Hallerback B, Ander S, Glise H. Effect of combined blockade of beta-adrenoceptors and acetylcholinesterase in the treatment of postoperative ileus after cholecystectomy. *Scand J Gastroenterol* 1987;22:420-424.

67. Ferraz AA, Wanderley GJ, Santos MA, Jr., Mathias CA, Araujo JG Jr, Ferraz EM. Effects of propranolol on human postoperative ileus. *Dig Surg* 2001; 18:305-310.

68. Henzi I, Walder B, Tramer MR. Metoclopramide in the prevention of postoperative nausea and vomiting: A quantitative systematic review of randomized, placebo-controlled studies. *Br J Anaesth* 1999;83:761-771.

69. Boeckxstaens GE, Pelckmans PA, Rampart M, Bogers JJ, Verbeuren TJ, Herman AG, Van Maercke YM. Pharmacological characterization of 5-hydroxy-tryptamine receptors in the canine terminal ileum and ileocolonic junction. *J Pharmacol Exp Ther* 1990;254:652-658.

70. Nagakura Y, Akuzawa S, Miyata K, Kamato T, Suzuki T, Ito H, Yamaguchi T. Pharmacological properties of a novel gastrointestinal prokinetic benzamide selective for human 5-HT4 receptor versus human 5-HT3 receptor. *Pharmacol Res* 1999;39:375-382.

71. Muller-Lissner SA, Fraas C, Hartl A. Cisapride offsets dopamine-induced slowing of fasting gastric emptying. *Digest Dis Sci* 1986;31:807-810.

72. Coremans G, Chaussade S, Janssens J, Vantrappen G. Stimulation of propulsive motility patterns by cisapride in the upper gut of man. *Digest Dis Sci* 1985;30:765.

73. Boghaert A, Haesaert G, Mourisse P, Verlinden M. Placebo-controlled trial of cisapride in postoperative ileus. *Acta Anaesthesiol Belg* 1987;38:195-199.

74. Verlinden M, Michiels G, Boghaert A, de Coster M, Dehertog P. Treatment of postoperative gastrointestinal atony. *Br J Surg* 1987;74:614-617.

75. Hallerback B, Bergman B, Bong H, Ekstrom P, Glise H, Lundgren K, Risberg O. Cisapride in the treatment of post-operative ileus. *Aliment Pharmacol Ther* 1991;5:503-511.

76. Carlsson L, Amos GJ, Andersson B, Drews L, Duker G, Wadstedt G. Electrophysiological characterization of the prokinetic agents cisapride and mo-

sapride in vivo and in vitro: Implications for proarrhythmic potential? *J Pharmacol Exp Ther* 1997;282:220-227.

77. Kii Y, Ito T. Effects of 5-HT4-receptor agonists, cisapride, mosapride citrate, and zacopride, on cardiac action potentials in guinea pig isolated papillary muscles. *J Cardiovasc Pharmacol* 1997;29:670-675.

78. Tonini M, De Ponti F, Di Nucci A, Crema F. Review article: Cardiac adverse effects of gastrointestinal prokinetics. *Aliment Pharmacol Ther* 1999;13:1585-1591.

79. Weber FH, Jr., Richards RD, McCallum RW. Erythromycin: A motilin agonist and gastrointestinal prokinetic agent. *Am J Gastroenterol* 1993;88:485-490.

80. Bungard TJ, Kale-Pradhan PB. Prokinetic agents for the treatment of postoperative ileus in adults: A review of the literature. *Pharmacotherapy* 1999;19:416-423.

81. Ruwart MJ, Klepper MS, Rush BD. Prostaglandin stimulation of gastrointestinal transit in post-operative ileus rats. *Prostaglandins* 1980;19:415-426.

82. Mulholland MW, Simeone DM. Prostaglandin E2 stimulation of acetylcholine release from guinea pig myenteric plexus neurons. *Am J Surg* 1993;166:552-556.

83. Yokoyama T, Kitazawa T, Takasaki K, Ishii A, Karasawa A. Recovery of gastrointestinal motility from post-operative ileus in dogs: Effects of Leu13-motilin (KW-5139) and prostaglandin F2 alpha. *Neurogastroenterol Motil* 1995;7:199-210.

84. Fanning J, Yu-Brekke S. Prospective trial of aggressive postoperative bowel stimulation following radical hysterectomy. *Gynecol Oncol* 1999;73:412-414.

85. Holdcroft A. Hormones and the gut. *Br J Anaesth* 2000;85:58-68.

86. Madsen PV, Lykkegaard-Nielsen M, Nielsen OV. Ceruletide reduces postoperative intestinal paralysis: A double-blind placebo-controlled trial. *Dis Colon Rectum* 1983;26:159-160.

87. Sadek SA, Cranford C, Eriksen C, Walker M, Campbell C, Baker PR, Wood RA, Cuschieri A. Pharmacological manipulation of adynamic ileus: Controlled randomized double-blind study of ceruletide on intestinal motor activity after elective abdominal surgery. *Aliment Pharmacol Ther* 1988;2:47-54.

88. Liu M, Wittbrodt E. Low-dose oral naloxone reverses opioid-induced constipation and analgesia. *J Pain Symptom Manage* 2002;23:48-53.

89. Bianchi G, Fiocchi R, Tavani A, Manara L. Quaternary narcotic antagonists' relative ability to prevent antinociception and gastrointestinal transit inhibition in morphine-treated rats as an index of peripheral selectivity. *Life Sci* 1982;30:1875-1883.

90. Russell J, Bass P, Goldberg LI, Schuster CR, Merz H. Antagonism of gut, but not central effects of morphine with quaternary narcotic antagonists. *Eur J Pharmacol* 1982;78:255-261.

91. Foss JF. A review of the potential role of methylnaltrexone in opioid bowel dysfunction. *Am J Surg* 2001;182:19S-26S.

92. Yuan CS, Foss JF, Osinski J, Toledano A, Roizen MF, Moss J. The safety and efficacy of oral methylnaltrexone in preventing morphine-induced delay in oral-cecal transit time. *Clin Pharmacol Ther* 1997;61:467-475.

93. Yuan CS, Foss JF, O'Connor M, Karrison T, Osinski J, Roizen MF, Moss J. Effects of enteric-coated methylnaltrexone in preventing opioid-induced delay in oral-cecal transit time. *Clin Pharmacol Ther* 2000;67:398-404.

94. Kurz A, Sessler DI. Opioid-induced bowel dysfunction: Pathophysiology and potential new therapies. *Drugs* 2003;63:649-671.

95. Schmidt WK. Alvimopan (ADL 8-2698) is a novel peripheral opioid antagonist. *Am J Surg* 2001;182:27S-38S.

96. Barr W, Nguyen P, Slattery M, R. R, Carpenter R. ADL 8-2698 reverses opioids induced delay in colonic transit. *Clin Pharmacol Ther* 2000;67:93.

97. Taguchi A, Sharma N, Saleem RM, Sessler DI, Carpenter RL, Seyedsadr M, Kurz A. Selective postoperative inhibition of gastrointestinal opioid receptors. *N Engl J Med* 2001;345:935-940.

98. Steinbrook RA. Epidural anesthesia and gastrointestinal motility. *Anesth Analg* 1998;86:837-844.

99. Rimback G, Cassuto J, Tollesson PO. Treatment of postoperative paralytic ileus by intravenous lidocaine infusion. *Anesth Analg* 1990;70:414-419.

100. Wallin G, Cassuto J, Hogstrom S, Rimback G, Faxen A, Tollesson PO. Failure of epidural anesthesia to prevent postoperative paralytic ileus. *Anesthesiology* 1986;65:292-297.

101. Scheinin B, Asantila R, Orko R. The effect of bupivacaine and morphine on pain and bowel function after colonic surgery. *Acta Anaesthesiol Scand* 1987; 31:161-164.

102. Ahn H, Bronge A, Johansson K, Ygge H, Lindhagen J. Effect of continuous postoperative epidural analgesia on intestinal motility. *Brit J Surg* 1988;75:1176-1178.

103. Wattwil M, Thoren T, Hennerdal S, Garvill JE. Epidural analgesia with bupivacaine reduces postoperative paralytic ileus after hysterectomy. *Anesth Analg* 1989;68:353-358.

104. Bredtmann RD, Herden HN, Teichmann W, Moecke HP, Kniesel B, Baetgen R, Tecklenburg A. Epidural analgesia in colonic surgery: Results of a randomized prospective study. *Brit J Surg* 1990;77:638-642.

105. Riwar A, Schar B, Grotzinger U. [Effect of continuous postoperative analgesia with peridural bupivacaine on intestinal motility following colorectal resection]. *Helv Chir Acta* 1992;58:729-733.

106. Liu SS, Carpenter RL, Mackey DC, Thirlby RC, Rupp SM, Shine TS, Feinglass NG, Metzger PP, Fulmer JT, Smith SL. Effects of perioperative analgesic technique on rate of recovery after colon surgery. *Anesthesiology* 1995;83:757-765.

107. de Leon-Casasola OA, Karabella D, Lema MJ. Bowel function recovery after radical hysterectomies: Thoracic epidural bupivacaine-morphine versus intravenous patient-controlled analgesia with morphine: A pilot study. *J Clin Anesth* 1996;8:87-92.

108. Neudecker J, Schwenk W, Junghans T, Pietsch S, Bohm B, Muller JM. Randomized controlled trial to examine the influence of thoracic epidural analgesia on postoperative ileus after laparoscopic sigmoid resection. *Br J Surg* 1999;86:1292-1295.

109. Carli F, Trudel JL, Belliveau P. The effect of intraoperative thoracic epidural anesthesia and postoperative analgesia on bowel function after colorectal surgery: A prospective, randomized trial. *Dis Colon Rectum* 2001;44:1083-1089.

110. Scott AM, Starling JR, Ruscher AE, DeLessio ST, Harms BA. Thoracic versus lumbar epidural anesthesia's effect on pain control and ileus resolution after restorative proctocolectomy. *Surgery* 1996;120:688-695; discussion 695-697.

111. Lewis KS, Han NH. Tramadol: A new centrally acting analgesic. *Am J Health Syst Pharm* 1997;54:643-652.

112. Scott LJ, Perry CM. Tramadol: A review of its use in perioperative pain. *Drugs* 2000;60:139-176.

113. Crighton IM, Martin PH, Hobbs GJ, Cobby TF, Fletcher AJ, Stewart PD. A comparison of the effects of intravenous tramadol, codeine, and morphine on gastric emptying in human volunteers. *Anesth Analg* 1998;87:445-449.

114. Elton C, Guest C, Pallett E, Rowbotham D. Effect of tramadol on gastric emptying of a liquid meal. *Br J Anaesth* 1999;82:471.

115. Wilder-Smith CH, Hill L, Wilkins J, Denny L. Effects of morphine and tramadol on somatic and visceral sensory function and gastrointestinal motility after abdominal surgery. *Anesthesiology* 1999;91:639-647.

116. Ferreira SH, Nakamura M, de Abreu Castro MS. The hyperalgesic effects of prostacyclin and prostaglandin E2. *Prostaglandins* 1978;16:31-37.

117. Furst DE, Minstrin T. Nonsteroidal antiinflammatory drugs; non opioid analgesics; drugs used in gout. In B Katzung (ed.), *Basic and clinical pharmacology.* East Norwalk, CT: McGraw Hill; 2001:596.

118. Pairet M, Ruckebusch Y. On the relevance of non-steroidal anti-inflammatory drugs in the prevention of paralytic ileus in rodents. *J Pharm Pharmacol* 1989;41:757-761.

119. Thor P, Konturek JW, Konturek SJ, Anderson JH. Role of prostaglandins in control of intestinal motility. *Am J Physiol* 1985;248:G353-G359.

120. Kelley MC, Hocking MP, Marchand SD, Sninsky CA. Ketorolac prevents postoperative small intestinal ileus in rats. *Am J Surg* 1993;165:107-111; discussion 112.

121. Cheng G, Cassissi C, Drexler PG, Vogel SB, Sninsky CA, Hocking MP. Salsalate, morphine, and postoperative ileus. *Am J Surg* 1996;171:85-88; discussion 88-89.

122. Gajraj NM. Cyclooxygenase-2 inhibitors. *Anesth Analg* 2003;96:1720-1738.

123. Gimbel JS, Brugger A, Zhao W, Verburg KM, Geis GS. Efficacy and tolerability of celecoxib versus hydrocodone/acetaminophen in the treatment of pain after ambulatory orthopedic surgery in adults. *Clin Ther* 2001;23:228-241.

124. Issioui T, Klein KW, White PF, Watcha MF, Coloma M, Skrivanek GD, Jones SB, Thornton KC, Marple BF. The efficacy of premedication with celecoxib and acetaminophen in preventing pain after otolaryngologic surgery. *Anesth Analg* 2002;94:1188-1193, table of contents.

125. Shen Q, Sinatra R. Preoperative rofecoxib 25mg, 50mg: Effects of postsurgical morphine consumption and effort dependent pain. *Anesthesiology* 2001;95:A961.

126. Schwarz NT, Kalff JC, Turler A, Engel BM, Watkins SC, Billiar TR, Bauer AJ. Prostanoid production via COX-2 as a causative mechanism of rodent postoperative ileus. *Gastroenterology* 2001;121:1354-1371.

127. Ruoff G, Lema M. Strategies in pain management: New and potential indications for COX-2 specific inhibitors. *J Pain Symptom Manage* 2003;25:S21-S31.

128. Fu ES, Miguel R, Scharf JE. Preemptive ketamine decreases postoperative narcotic requirements in patients undergoing abdominal surgery. *Anesth Analg* 1997;84:1086-1090.

Chapter 8

Postsurgical Bowel Dysfunction in the Gynecologic Patient

Eric J. Bieber

INTRODUCTION

In spite of the change to approaching many gynecologic conditions in a minimally invasive manner, many surgeries are still being performed via open laparotomy. Hysterectomy remains one of the most commonly performed procedures in the United States, with more than a half million cases performed annually. Although there has been a push to perform more hysterectomies via a laparoscopic or vaginal approach, the majority of these cases are still performed in a standard open manner.

The substantial morbidity associated with such procedures is well-known. One of the most common issues is lack of return of normal bowel activity and the associated prolongation of inpatient hospitalization. Gastrointestinal issues such as obstipation, constipation, diarrhea, and abdominal and pelvic pain, associated with both the primary surgery as well as the underlying abnormalities of bowel dysfunction induced by the surgery, are the source of a significant reduction in quality of life (QOL), both in the immediate as well as in prolonged recovery periods. While all such issues are well-known to all practicing gynecologists, there has been little discussion of such issues or substantive research to evaluate methods for improving outcomes in this area. Much of the published literature is not evidence based, nor are many of the recommendations and tenets that we were taught during our training. Current dogma recognizes that cost efficacy is more than just the reduction in hospital days that may be associated with any practice change; it is also the impact on the patient's function when she is at home and how quickly the patient might return to normal activity and, as such, function as a member of society. Such issues are not mundane in that patients and employers suffer significant losses when patients are absent from work or are unable to adequately function in their jobs.

This chapter reviews the pathophysiologic events associated with laparotomy and major gynecologic surgery. Current data regarding both short- and long-term gastrointestinal dysfunction after gynecologic surgery are reviewed. More recent evidenced-based data regarding timing of first feeding as well as the impact and necessity of nasogastric (NG) suction are discussed. The impact of various forms of anesthesia on return of bowel function are also presented. Finally, interesting data regarding opioid antagonist treatment and the potential for novel investigation are described relative to gynecologic surgery.

PATHOPHYSIOLOGY

All surgeons have had to deal with the issue of impaired bowel and gastrointestinal function after laparotomy. Numerous investigations have been performed over the past six decades to evaluate the underlying etiology of physiologic dysfunction after surgery. It was believed that the handling of the bowel during surgery contributed to some dysmotility, while more recent data has focused on the role of opioid receptors and their impact on bowel myoelectric activity. In addition, open gynecologic surgery has been associated with high rates of postoperative nausea and vomiting, approaching 50 to 75 percent of all patients and profoundly impacting patient perception of QOL after surgery.[1,2]

In 1975, Wilson presented very interesting data that conflicted with some prior long-held tenets of surgery.[3] They used radiotelemetry capsules to measure intralumenal pressures and the location of the capsules in the GI tract of postoperative patients. They noted that while pressure changes in the colon suggested return of some myolectric activity after surgery, these contractions might not be functional in appropriate propulsion and forward sequencing of enteric contents. In this study, there was no impact of duration of surgery on return of bowel function and this occurred on average after 40 to 48 hours (see Table 8.1). In the study conducted by Woods and colleagues, electromechanical bowel function was evaluated in slump-tail monkeys.[4] They noted a limited effect of general anesthesia and laparotomy on both antral and small bowel function, whereas right colonic activity was suppressed for 24 hours and sigmoid colon contractile activity was suppressed for 72 hours. Table 8.2 and Figure 8.1 demonstrate the differential response of the various GI segments to myoelectric contraction suppression after the inciting event.

Studies of gastric function suggest that without feedings, the stomach secretes 500 to 1,000 cc of fluid per day with equivalent amounts being secreted by the pancreas.[5] While the initial focus for reducing postoperative ileus was on limiting surgical manipulation of bowel and decreasing the amount of fluid presented to the small intestine, newer data suggest stimulation of opioid receptors is also involved and plays a role in suppression of bowel activity.[6] Current thought

TABLE 8.1. The effect of length of operation on the return of colonic motility.

Length of operation (hours)	Average time taken for return of pressure activity (hours)	Average time elapsing before first passage of flatus (hours)	Average time taken for passage of 80 percent of markers (days)	Average time for visible colonic decompression on radiographs (days)
1-2	55	65	6	4
2-3	42	57	5	5
3-4	39	70	7	5

Source: Wilson JP. Postoperative motility of the large intestine in man. *Gut* 1975;16(9):689-692. Reprinted with permission from the BMJ Publishing Group.

TABLE 8.2. Summary of bowel response to ileus operation.

	Before operation	Hours After Operation			Hours elapsing to normal
		2	15	24	
Antrum	7.1 ± 1.5	4.8 ± 10	13.3 ± 3.8	13.3 ± 10.0	8
Small bowel	124 ± 14	72 ± 31	136.0 ± 29	134.0 ± 82.5	7
Right colon	34.8 ± 3.4	$7.3 \pm 3.5^{**}$	$21.9 \pm 4.2^{*}$	$22.9 \pm 6.0^{*}$	48
Sigmoid colon	38.8 ± 2.8	$4.1 \pm 1.7^{**}$	$22.6 \pm 4.5^{**}$	$24.0 \pm 10.0^{**}$	72

Notes: Contractions per hour, mean ± one standard deviation ($n = 11$).
Source: Reprinted from *Surgery,* 84(4), Woods JH, Erikson LW, Condon RE, Schulte WJ, Sillin LF, Postoperative ileus: A colonic problem? 527-533, Copyright 1978, with permission from Elsevier.
$^{*}p < 0.05$.
$^{**}p < 0.01$.

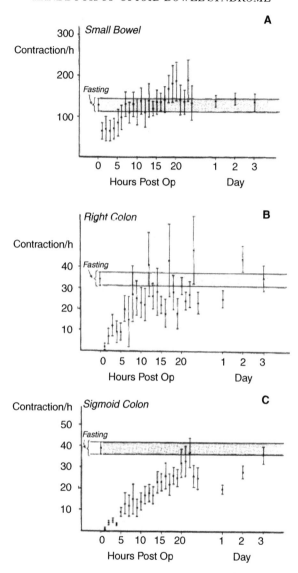

FIGURE 8.1. Gut response to ileus operation. The shaded bar represents the mean ± one standard error (SE) of fasting contractions during baseline measurements. Each point is the mean ± one SE of postoperative contractile activity, where *n* = 11. *Source:* Reprinted from *Surgery,* 84(4), Woods JH, Erikson LW, Condon RE, Schulte WJ, Sillin LF, Postoperative ileus: A colonic problem? 527-533, Copyright 1978, with permission from Elsevier.

suggests a two-pathway source of stimulation of opioid receptors in surgical patients—initially through the endogenous release of opioids from surgical stress and later the use of exogenous opioids during and after surgery for pain management. Frantzides et al. have demonstrated that morphine sulfate inhibits the mesenteric plexus from releasing acetylcholine.[7] Predictably, this action increases colonic tone while decreasing propulsive force and likely contributes to delays in return of bowel activity.

BOWEL FUNCTION AFTER HYSTERECTOMY

There have been questions regarding the long-term impact of hysterectomy on subsequent bowel function. Unfortunately, few well-done trials exist to provide us with data in counseling and following patients. The concept that through the process of performing a simple or radical hysterectomy we affect the neurologic or structural integrity so as to create bowel dysfunction does not at present appear to be born out by data. One difficulty in evaluating nonprospective data is the relatively high incidence of irritable bowel syndrome (IBS) in gynecologic patients.[8] This is consistent with data from Clarke et al. who noted that 19 percent of patients reporting constipation prior to total abdominal hysterectomy and 16 percent reporting symptoms after the surgery.[9] Similarly, Prior et al. reported that more than 20 percent of patients preoperatively had IBS symptoms. Interestingly, 60 percent had symptom resolution with hysterectomy but 5 percent of nonsymptomatic patients had a new onset of IBS after surgery.[10] The Maine Women's Health Study similarly noted no significant change in bowel function after hysterectomy.[11] Gurnari also retrospectively evaluated patients undergoing radical versus simple hysterectomy and noted no significant change with the latter after surgery but an increase in new onset constipation and loss of urge with radical hysterectomy.[12]

In an interesting questionnaire study, Weber and colleagues queried 43 females by questionnaire before and one year following total abdominal hysterectomy.[13] In this study, unfortunately 71 percent of patients' primary indication for surgery was myomata. It is possible that large myomata may create their own symptomatology from pressure, which could impact results. Figure 8.2 demonstrates a trend to-

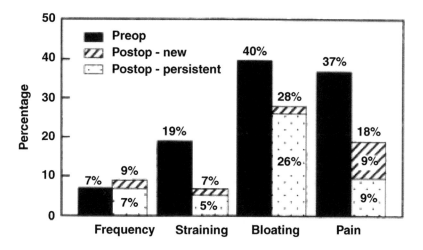

FIGURE 8.2. Lower gastrointestinal symptoms in 43 women before and after abdominal hysterectomy. No changes were statistically significant. Abnormal frequency of bowel movements was defined as less than every other day. For other symptoms of straining, bloating, and pain (abdominal pain or gas cramps), percentage reflects proportion of women with each symptom more than once a week. *Source:* Reprinted from *American Journal of Obstetrics and Gynecology,* 181, Weber AM, Walters MD, Schover LR, Church JM, Piedmonte MR, Functional outcomes and satisfaction after abdominal hysterectomy, 530-535, Copyright 1999, with permission from Elsevier.

ward decreased symptoms of straining, bloating, and pain after surgery, however, none were statistically significant. Of note, these symptoms are common both before and after surgery. Yet there seems to be little suggestion of a profound negative change with surgery.

In an interesting trial from the United Kingdom, Roy and co-workers evaluated three groups of patients with constipation who were undergoing biofeedback: one group with no prior surgery, one group of patients posthysterectomy with no change after surgery, and one group of patients whose constipation was worsened or precipitated by hysterectomy.[14] Patients improved similarly in all three groups, leading the authors to hypothesize that reversible factors and not neural or structural damage may be responsible for the symptoms.

There does exist opportunity for future studies to more specifically address differences between radical and simple hysterectomy, as well as long-term results. Carlson, in summarizing these issues, states, "The existing evidence suggests that hysterectomy rarely has any clinical significant adverse effects on bowel and bladder function."[15]

EFFECT OF EARLY FEEDINGS AND NG USE ON BOWEL FUNCTION

Standard surgical dogma for years dictated that diet should be advanced based on evidence of return of bowel function, in other words, decreased NG output, increased bowel sounds, passage of flatus, and bowel movement. Historically, surgeons have been slow to advance patients from liquid to soft to full diet. Recently, the entire paradigm of diet management in the postoperative time period has been called into question. Interestingly, managing patients in the standard manner that we were taught may have contributed to GI slowdown.

The basis for slowly returning patients to a standard diet was based on the assumption that early feeding might increase nausea or emesis and lead to aspiration, and increased pressure on fascia, skin closures, and anastomosis in the case of bowel reanastomosis. We also wrongly believed that by withholding oral intake, we were actually promoting quicker GI recovery and thus decreasing length of stay and improving QOL parameters. Many of us were also taught to use NG suctioning after difficult surgery. It appears that this latter issue has undergone change in recent years. In a survey sent to members of the Society of Gynecologic Oncology, 3 percent of respondents reported routine NG suction in only 15 percent of total abdominal hysterectomies, 29 percent of radical hysterectomies, and 34 percent of patients after retroperitoneal lymph node dissection.[16] However, the majority of surgeons (80 to 90 percent) continue to use NG suction after large or small bowel resection. Cutillo et al. randomized 122 patients who underwent laparotomy for gynecologic malignancy, but who did not have bowel resection, into an early feeding arm with no NG suction and clear liquid diet on postoperative day 1, advanced to semiliquid, then as tolerated versus standard NG suctions until flatus or low NG output.[17] Patients in the "quick feed" group had statistically and clinically significant decreases in resolution of ileus, first passage of stools, and decreased length of stay. Both groups had similar rates of nausea and emesis, and only 10 percent of patients in the early feed group required subsequent NG placement.

Pearl and his group performed a randomized controlled trial of 200 patients undergoing laparotomy for gynecologic malignancy, evaluating clear liquid diet on postoperative day 1 and advanced as tolerated versus NPO until return of bowel function.[18] While nausea was higher in the early feeding group (43.5 versus 24.3 percent), substantial decreases were again noted in the time taken to develop bowel sounds, initiation of clear and regular diet, and hospital length of stay (LOS). Major complications were the same for each group as were emesis and abdominal distension and patients in each group who tolerated either clear or solid feedings on the first attempt (see Table 8.3).

Data have also recently been published with general gynecologic patients. MacMillian et al. randomly assigned 139 women undergoing either major vaginal or abdominal gynecologic surgery to an early feeding of a low residue diet six hours postoperatively versus traditional management of clear liquids with bowel sounds and regular diet with flatus.[19] The number of patients with ileus was 3.0 percent for the early group and 5.8 percent for the late feeding group, and this difference was statistically significant. Other than the late group reporting more nausea, no other differences were seen. Similarly, Steed and her group prospectively randomized patients having major abdominal gynecologic surgery to a standard feeding protocol versus clear liquids on postoperative day 1 and at the point of tolerance of 500 cc of clear liquids, advancement of the diet.[20] In this Canadian study, LOS decreased by two days to 4.0 in the early feeding group and no differences were seen in ileus, emesis, or other complications between the two groups. Figure 8.3 demonstrates the decreased LOS in the early group and although U.S. patients may be discharged more expeditiously, the finding of patient tolerance to early feeding remains consistent with other studies.

Schilder et al. similarly randomized patients to traditional management versus clear liquid postoperative day 1 and advancement with tolerance of 500 cc.[21] Their study group was composed of both oncologic and nononcologic gynecology patients having major abdominal surgery. A noteworthy difference was an increase in the incidence of emesis in the early feeding group. In this American trial, LOS also statistically decreased from 4.02 to 3.12 days.

TABLE 8.3. Clear liquid diet on postoperative day 1 and advanced as tolerated versus NPO until return of bowel function.

| | Group | | |
| | Early | Traditional | |
Category	(*N* = 92)	(*N* = 103)	*P*
Morbidity			
Nausea	43.5	24.3	.006
Vomiting	5.3	4.2	NS
Abdominal distention	40.2	35.9	NS
Nasogastric tube use	3.3	6.7	NS
Duration (d)	2.7 ± 0.6	3.1 ± 1.3	NS
Diet tolerance on first attempt			
Clear liquid diet	86.8	91.3	NS
If intolerant, time to tolerance (d)	2.6 ± 1.8	4.1± 2.1	NS
Regular diet	89.0	95.2	NS
If intolerant, time to tolerance (d)	3.6 ± 1.9	5.0 ± 2.5	NS
Intervals			
Bowel sounds	1.8 ± 1.2	2.3 ± 1.2	.007
Flatus	3.2 ± 1.5	3.6 ± 1.4	NS
Clear liquid diet	1.2 ± 1.1	3.5 ± 1.5	<.0001
Regular diet	2.3 ± 1.4	4.2 ± 1.5	<.0001
Hospital stay	4.6 ± 2.1	5.8 ± 2.7	.001

Note: Data are presented as mean ± standard deviation, or percent; NS = not significant. *Source:* Reprinted from *Obstetrics and Gynecology,* 92, Pearl ML, Valea FA, Fischer M, Mahler L, Chalas E, A randomized controlled trial of early postoperative feeding in gynecologic oncology patients undergoing intra-abdominal surgery, 94-97, Copyright 1998, with permission from American College of Obstetricians and Gynecologists.

Fanning and Yu-Brekke have recently published two trials attempting to aggressively stimulate bowel function to improve early GI function and allow discharge. In the first trial, 20 patients who underwent radical hysterectomy began with 30 cc milk of magnesia (MOM) b.i.d. on postoperative day 1 and bicolic suppositories QD starting on postoperative day 2.[22] Patients began a clear diet after fla-

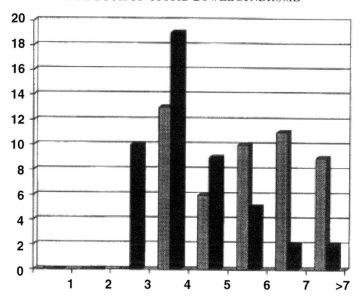

FIGURE 8.3. Length of hospital stay distribution in days, group A versus group B ($P = .0001$). The x-axis indicates the hospital day of discharge; the y-axis indicates the number of patients. The gray bars indicate group A (traditional feeding); the black bars indicate group B (early feeding). *Source:* Reprinted from *American Journal of Obstetrics and Gynecology,* 186, Steed HL, Capstick V, Flood C, Schepansky A, Schulz J, Mayes DC, A randomized controlled trial of early versus "traditional" postoperative oral intake after major abdominal gynecological surgery, 861-865, Copyright 2002, with permission from Elsevier.

tus or bowel movement and were discharged 12 hours after starting the clear liquid diet. Diet was then advanced at home. When they compared time of discharge to their prior trial, there was a 50 percent reduction. However, it is unclear what role the MOM and suppositories had in facilitating GI function. In the second trial, patients who underwent radical hysterectomy began a clear liquid diet and oral 66 percent sodium phosphate solution (Fleet Phospho Soda) on postoperative day 1. Patients were discharged with flatus or stool, which averaged three to five days.[23] In these noncomparative studies there seems to be a decrease in time in the onset of bowel function. However, larger prospective randomized trials will provide better evidence for efficacy of any of these treatments.

EPIDURALS, GENERAL ANESTHESIA,
AND PATIENT-CONTROLLED ANALGESIA

There are relatively limited investigations comparing either intra-operative versus postoperative regimens for anesthesia or pain control in the gynecologic population and the subsequent impact on bowel function. Early data had suggested that epidural anesthesia was not effectual in decreasing the incidence of ileus after surgery.[24] However, more recent data using modern techniques suggest use of epidurals with nonopioids may improve outcomes.

Callesen and colleagues evaluated 40 patients undergoing total abdominal hysterectomy and randomly assigned patients to epidural/spinal versus general anesthesia.[25] Postoperatively, both groups had epidurals for pain control. The group that received general anesthesia had epidurals with bupivacaine and morphine sulfate, and the group that had epidurals used for primary anesthesia continued using bupivacaine. Patients who had general anesthesia had lower rates of pain after surgery but higher nausea and vomiting scores. They also received fewer doses of subsequent supplemental opioids. Return of bowel function was noted to be similar in both groups but with a trend toward earlier return in the nongeneral anesthesia group. Similarly, Thoren et al. evaluated 22 patients having hysterectomies under general anesthesia who were treated with postoperative epidural morphine or bupivicaine.[26] Consistent with others, they noted a prolonged period of recovery of normal bowel function of 92 hours in the morphine group versus 57 hours in the bupivicaine group.

An interesting Canadian trial evaluated the use of postoperative patient-controlled analgesia (PCA) versus intramuscular opioids in patients after hysterectomy.[27] In this large prospective study of 126 patients, they surprisingly found comparable analgesia, with markedly reduced costs by not using PCA. Consistent with the fact that both used opioids, there were no differences in speed to discharge, resumption of liquid or solid diet, or flatus. An interesting editorial disagreed strongly with the protocol and ability to generalize the data to a postoperative population.[28]

OPIOID ANTAGONISTS

It is currently believed that besides surgical stimulation of the bowel during the manipulation that invariably occurs with surgery, opioid stimulation through both central release and exogenous administration also impacts the development of postoperative ileus.[6] In interesting studies, both Frantzides and Cali et al. have evaluated the impact of opioids such as morphine sulfate and found delays in return of colonic activity and prolongation of ileus.[7,29] As surgeons, this creates the dilemma of knowing that one of the most commonly used agents for postoperative pain may be acting in a negative fashion by inherently decreasing bowel activity and prolonging our patients' stays and recoveries.

Several investigators have attempted to use opioid antagonists such as naloxone to impact bowel dysfunction associated with opioid use.[30-32] Generally, these studies have been performed in patients who chronically use opioid agents. Although such trials have been effective, nalaxone given orally may be sufficiently absorbed to precipitate withdrawal or increase pain in chronic opioid users.[32]

More recently a selective opioid antagonist, ADL 8-2698 (alvimopan), has been investigated. Interestingly, it is poorly absorbed through the gut but is long acting and orally effective.[33] Initial clinical studies were performed in patients undergoing dental surgery.[34] In this trial they were able to document the lack of substantive impact of the drug on opioid anesthesia and analgesia. These trials led to a pilot clinical trial of the agent in patients undergoing either partial colectomy ($N = 15$) or simple and radical abdominal hysterectomy ($N = 63$).[35] Patients were randomly assigned to placebo, 1 mg, or 6 mg of ADL 8-2698. Unfortunately, the data were presented in an aggregated fashion, and the results relative to only the hysterectomy patients were not reported. Figure 8.4 demonstrates the decreased time to first flatus, first bowel movement, and discharge, which were all statistically decreased in placebo versus the 6 mg dose. Time to flatus was decreased from 70 to 49 hours, bowel movement from 111 to 70 hours, and discharge from hospital was decreased from 91 to 68 hours. These changes are likely not only statistically significant but also clinically relevant. Equally important, Table 8.4 also demonstrates the lack of impact of either dose on patient pain scores or their

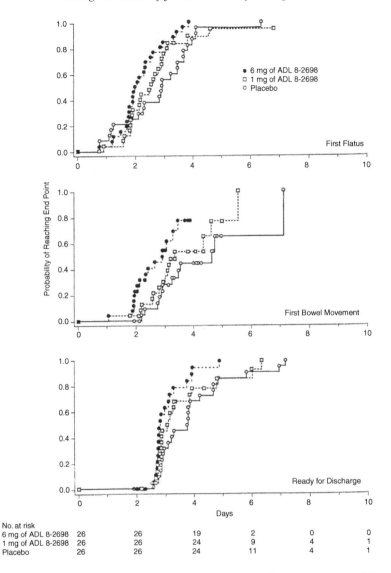

No. at risk					
6 mg of ADL 8-2698	26	26	19	2	0	0
1 mg of ADL 8-2698	26	26	24	9	4	1
Placebo	26	26	24	11	4	1

FIGURE 8.4. Kaplan-Meier estimates of the primary efficacy outcomes of time to first passage of flatus, time to first bowel movement, and time until patient was ready for discharge. *Source:* Taguchi A, Sharma N, Saleem RM, Sessler DI, Carpenter RL, Seyedsadr M, Kurz A. Selective postoperative inhibition of gastrointestinal opioid receptors. *N Eng J Med* 2001; 345: 935-940. Copyright © 2001 Massachussetts Medical Society. All rights reserved.

TABLE 8.4. Postoperative consumption of morphine, adverse effects, and median times to outcomes.

Variable	Placebo (N = 26)	1 mg of ADL 8-2698 (N = 26)	6 mg of ADL 8-2698 (N = 26)	P Value[a]
	Mean SD			
Cumulative morphine sulfate (mg)	71 ± 58	70 ± 61	71 ± 52	0.91
Maximal pain (mm)[b]	54 ± 25	62 ± 24	53 ± 21	0.30
Maximal nausea (mm)[b]	38 ± 28	38 ± 33	18 ± 26	0.02
Maximal itching (mm)[b]	16 ± 28	25 ± 29	28 ± 36	0.48
Maximal abdominal cramping (mm)[b]	30 ± 29	38 ± 31	21 ± 24	0.13
	Median (interquartile range)			
Time to first passage of flatus (hr)	70 (48-88)	61 (46-72)	49 (43-63)	0.03
Time to first bowel movement (hr)	111 (70-171)	80 (67-111)	70 (50-83)	0.01
Time to first liquids (hr)	38 (26-60)	30 (21-41)	26 (18-40)	0.14
Time to first solids (hr)	92 (69-112)	69 (64-93)	59 (52-68)	<0.001
Time until ready for discharge (hr)	91 (70-112)	74 (67-94)	68 (65-68)	0.03
Time until actual discharge (hr)	100 (79-121)	93 (75-118)	71 (56-89)	<0.001

[a]P values refer to differences among the three groups. The morphine doses include the morphine-equivalent doses of meperidine hydrochloride (7.5 mg of meperidine equals 1.0 mg of morphine).
[b]Values were measured on a visual-analog scale.
Source: Taguchi A, Sharma N, Saleem RM, Sessler DI, Carpenter RL, Seyedsadr M, Kurz A. Selective postoperative inhibition of gastrointestinal opioid receptors. N Eng J Med 2001;345:935-940. Copyright © 2001 Massachussetts Medical Society. All rights reserved.

use of narcotic. Patients at the 6 mg dose were also noted to tolerate oral intake sooner with less nausea and emesis.

These results have led to multiple additional clinical trials with this agent, as well as created greater interest in the prospect of identifying additional compounds with similar attributes. Our improved understanding of the location and identity of novel opioid receptors in the gut and our pharmacologic ability to manipulate them (as discussed in other chapters) will likely lead to further improvements in our ability to use opioid agents without the risk of adversely affecting bowel function.

CONCLUSIONS

The problem of bowel dysfunction after major abdominal and especially gynecologic surgery remains unresolved. While the issue was studied for the better part of the twentieth century, there remains limited modalities for treatment other than time. It is surprising that as surgeons we continue to use such methods as NG suction or continuing patients NPO for extended periods of time, which are not founded in evidence-based medicine. There may still be a place in some clinical situations, but review of the data suggests that in the majority of gynecologic patients we are actually not helping patient recovery by using these methodologies. The reader is thus directed to the citations in this chapter to review and consider how these revelations might impact management.

The finding of selective peripheral opioid antagonists is very exciting.[33-37] These early clinical trial results should encourage scientists to press forward in the quest toward improved analgesia in the postoperative time period without the unfortunate sequelae of bowel dysfunction and immobility. These findings bode well for further opportunities to aid our patients in having little or no pain after surgery and returning to a normal quality of life as quickly as possible.

NOTES

1. Hovorka J, Kortilla K, Erkolo O. Nausea and vomiting after general anaesthesia with isoflurone, enflurane or fentanyl in combination with nitrous oxide and oxygen. *Eur J Anaesthesiol* 1988;5:177-182.

2. Madej TH, Simpson KH. Comparison of the use of domperidone, droperidol and metoclopramide in the prevention of nausea and vomiting following major gynaecological surgery. *Br J Anaesth* 1986;58:884-887.

3. Wilson JP. Postoperative motility of the large intestine in man. *Gut* 1975; 16(9):689-692.

4. Woods JH, Erickson LW, Condon RE, Schulte WJ, Sillin LF. Postoperative ileus: A colonic problem? *Surgery* 1978;84(4):527-533.

5. Bufo AJ, Feldman S, Daniels GA, Liberman RC. Early postoperative feeding. *Dis Col Rectum* 1994;37:584-589.

6. Holte K, Kehlet H. Postoperative ileus a preventable event. *Br J Surg* 2000; 87:1480-1493.

7. Frantzides CT, Cowles V, Salaymeh B, Tekin E, Condon RE. Morphine effects on human colonic myoelectric activity in the postoperative period. *Am J Surg* 1992;163:144-149.

8. Prior A, Wilson R, Whorwell PJ, Faragher EB. Irritable bowel syndrome in the gynecological clinic. *Dig Dis Sci* 1989;34:1820-1824.

9. Clarke A, Black N, Rowe P, Mott S, Howle K. Indication for and outcome of total abdominal hysterectomy for benign disease: A prospective cohort study. *Br J Obstet Gynaecol* 1995;102:611-620.

10. Prior A, Stanley KM, Smith ARB, Read NW. Relation between hysterectomy and the irritable bowel: A prospective study. *Gut* 1992;33:814-817.

11. Carleson KJ, Miller BA, Fowler FJ. The Maine Women's Health Study: I. Outcomes of hysterectomy. *Obstet Gynecol* 1994;83:556-565.

12. Gurnari M, Mazziotti F, Corazziari E. Chronic constipation after gynecological surgery: A retrospective study. *Ital J Gastroenterol* 1988;20:183-186.

13. Weber AM, Walters MD, Schover LR, Church JM, Piedmonte MR. Functional outcomes and satisfaction after abdominal hysterectomy. *Am J Obstet Gynecol* 1999;181:530-535.

14. Roy AJ, Emmanuel AV, Storrie JB, Bowers J, Kamm MA. Behavioral treatment (biofeedback) for constipation following hysterectomy. *Br J Surg* 1999; 87:100-105.

15. Carlson KJ. Outcomes of hysterectomy. *Clin Obstet Gynecol* 1997;40:939-946.

16. Brewer MA, Bodurka DC, Bevers M, Gershenson DM, Burke TM, Wolk JK. Postoperative nasogastric intubation in gynecologic oncology patients: A survey. *Gynecol Oncol* 1998;68:126.

17. Cutillo G, Maneschi F, Franchi M, Giannice R, Scambia G, Benedetti-Panici P. Early feeding compared with nasogastric decompression after major oncologic surgery: A randomized study. *Obstet Gynecol* 1999;93:41-45.

18. Pearl ML, Valea FA, Fischer M, Mahler L, Chalas E. A randomized controlled trial of early postoperative feeding in gynecologic oncology patients undergoing intra-abdominal surgery. *Obstet Gynecol* 1998;92:94-97.

19. MacMillan SL, Kammerer-Doak D, Rogers RG, Parker KM. Early feeding and the incidence of gastrointestinal symptoms after major gynecologic surgery. *Obstet Gynecol* 2000;96:604-608.

20. Steed HL, Capstick V, Flood C, Schepansky A, Schulz J, Mayes DC. A randomized controlled trial of early versus "traditional" postoperative oral intake after major abdominal gynecologic surgery. *Am J Obstet Gynecol* 2002:186:861-865.

21. Schilder JM, Hurteau JA, Look KY, Moore DH, Raff G, Stehman FB, Sutton GP. A prospective controlled trial of early postoperative oral intake following major abdominal gynecologic surgery. *Gynecol Oncol* 1997;67:235-240.

22. Fanning J, Yu-Brekke S. Prospective trial of aggressive postoperative bowel stimulation following radical hysterectomy. *Gynecol Oncol* 1999;73:412-414.

23. Kraus K. Fanning J. Prospective trial of early feeding and bowel stimulation after radical hysterectomy. *Am J Obstet Gynecol* 2000;182:996-998.

24. Wallin G, Cassuto J, Hostrom S, Rimback G, Faxen A, Tollesson PO. Failure of epidural anesthesia to prevent postoperative paralytic ileus. *Anesthesiology* 1986; 65:292-297.

25. Callesen T, Schouenborg L, Nielsen D, Guldager H, Kehlet H. Combined epidural-spinal opioid-free anaesthesia and analgesia for hysterectomy. *Br J Anesth* 1999;82:881-885.

26. Thoren T, Sundberg A, Wattwil M, Garvill JE, Jurgensen U. Effects of epidural bupivacaine and epidural morphine on bowel function and pain after hysterectomy. *Acta Anaesthesiol Scand* 1989;33:181-185.

27. Choiniere M, Rittenhouse BE, Perreault S, Chartrand D, Rousseau P, Smith B, Pepler C. Efficacy and costs of patient-controlled analgesia versus regularly administered intramuscular opioid therapy. *Anesthesiology* 1998;89:1377-1388.

28. Fitzgibbon DR, Ready LB, Ching JM. Intramuscular opioid injections: A step in the wrong direction. *Anesthesiology* 1999;91:891-892.

29. Cali RL, Meade PG, Swanson MS, Freeman C. Effect of morphine and incision length on bowel function after colectomy. *Dis Colon Rectum* 2000;43:163-168.

30. Meissner W, Schmidt U, Hartmann M, Kath R, Reinhart K. Oral naloxone reverses opioid-associated constipation. *Pain* 2000;84:105-109.

31. Culpepper-Morgan JA, Inturrisi CE, Portenoy RK, Foley K, Houde RW, Marsh F, Kreek MJ. Treatment of opioid induced constipation with oral naloxone: A pilot study. *Clin Pharmacol Ther* 1992;52:90-95.

32. Sykes NP. An investigation of the ability of oral naloxone to correct opioid-related constipation in patients with advanced cancer. *Palliat Med* 1996;10:135-144.

33. Zimmerman DM, Gidda JS, Cantrell BE, Schoepp DD, Johnson BG, Leander JD. Discovery of a potent, peripherally selective trans-3,4-dimethyl-4-(3-hydroxyphenyl) piperidine opioid antagonist for the treatment of gastrointestinal mobility disorders. *J Med Chem* 1994;37:2262-2265.

34. Liu SS, Hodgson PS, Carpenter RL, Fricke JR Jr. ADL8-2698, a trans-3,4-dimethyl-4-(3-hydroxyphenyl) piperidine prevents gastrointestinal effects of intravenous morphine without affecting analgesia. *Clin Pharmacol Ther* 2001;69:66-71.

35. Taguchi A, Sharma N, Saleem RM, Sessler DI, Carpenter RL, Seyedsadr M, Kurz A. Selective postoperative inhibition of gastrointestinal opioid receptors. *N Engl J Med* 2001;345:935-940.

36. Yuan CS, Foss JF, O'Connor M, Toledano A, Roizen MF, Moss J. Methylnaltrexone prevents morphine-induced delay in oral-fecal transit time without affecting analgesia: A double-blind randomized placebo-controlled trial. *Clin Pharmacol Ther* 1996;59:469-475.

37. Yuan CS, Foss JF, O'Connor M, Osinski J, Karrison T, Moss J, Roizen MF. Methylnaltrexone for reversal of constipation due to chronic methadone use: A randomized, controlled trial. *JAMA* 2000;283:367-372.

SECTION III:
ADVANCES IN TREATING
OPIOID BOWEL DYSFUNCTION

Chapter 9

Using Oral Naloxone in Management of Opioid Bowel Dysfunction

Nigel P. Sykes

Opioid bowel dysfunction principally gives rise either to constipation or to nausea and vomiting. Although intravenous naloxone has been used with success in one study of the control of opioid-related emesis,[1] the applications of oral naloxone have been in the management of constipation associated with opioid analgesia.

For naloxone to control constipation without reversing the analgesia that the opioid is usually intended to provide, two conditions must be met. First, the constipating effect of opioids must be mediated at least predominantly peripherally, in separation from the central analgesic actions of these drugs. Second, it must be possible for naloxone to act peripherally while leaving the central actions of the opioid intact.

EVIDENCE FOR A PERIPHERAL SITE OF OPIOID CONSTIPATING ACTION

Detailed investigation of opioid actions on the gut is complicated by species differences and by the likelihood that responses depend on the state of activity of the intestine at the time. Margolin[2] found that intestinal transit was slowed in mice after intracerebroventricular injections of morphine at doses considerably lower than those effective intravenously, a finding confirmed in other animal species.[3,4] Selective opioid receptor studies have indicated that central nervous system (CNS) mediation of gastrointestinal transit occurs not only at the cerebral level but also in the spinal cord.[5]

However, there is also evidence of the importance of direct intestinal effects of opioids even in rodents and certainly in man. The ability of intraperitoneal morphine to slow gut transit in the rat is inhibited by the quaternary opioid antagonist diallylnalorphine, which had no effect on transit slowing induced by a similar dose of morphine delivered intracranially.[6] The significance of this result is that quaternary derivatives of opioid antagonists do not readily cross the blood-brain barrier and their actions are thus assumed to be peripheral rather than central. In addition, higher morphine concentrations are found in the intestine after peripheral administration than in the brain,[7] suggesting that a peripheral site of action is important. Crucially, the denervated bowel continues to show response to systemic opioids, indicating that although centrally mediated constipating effects of opioids exist, it is the peripheral mechanisms that are fundamental.[8]

Loperamide is an opioid agonist that has achieved therapeutic success as an antidiarrheal. This is because it is effective at slowing intestinal hurry while displaying very low levels of other opioid effects, at least in adults.[9] The oral bioavailability of loperamide is around 1 percent and this presumably allows it to have a peripheral constipating effect without giving rise to analgesia or mental effects. In light of this evidence, it seems likely that at least a major component of opioid-induced constipation is mediated peripherally. If central and peripheral actions can be separated for an opioid agonist such as loperamide, there is the possibility that they could also be separated for an opioid antagonist.

NALOXONE AS AN OPIOID ANTAGONIST

Naloxone is derived by the substitution of an allyl group for the *N*-methyl group in oxymorphone. It is a competitive antagonist of opioid receptors within and without the central nervous system. When given to humans who are not taking opioids, it causes only mild drowsiness even at doses of 24 mg. It does not cause diarrhea in such individuals but may significantly alter intestinal motility.

The principal clinical use of naloxone is as a treatment of morphine overdose, and for this purpose it is given intravenously. Its established oral use is in combination with methadone to reduce the risk of parenteral methadone abuse in drug withdrawal programs.[10] It has been found possible to produce and maintain an opioid blockade using oral naloxone, but doses of 2 or 3 g may be required.

The reason for this is that although naloxone is rapidly absorbed by mouth, nearly all of an ingested dose is metabolized in the first hepatic transit. This is achieved by glucuronidation, which can also occur in the gut mucosa. The metabolite is presumed to be inactive, but it can be broken down by intestinal bacteria to yield the native molecule again. However, as a result of this pattern of metabolism, the oral bioavailability of naloxone in humans is only about 3 percent.[11] A 30 mg dose of naloxone given systemically produced a peak plasma level of 80 ng/mL, whereas the same dose orally gave a level of only 3.6 ng/mL.[12] Excretion of naloxone is renal and its plasma half-life is approximately 120 minutes.

Naloxone can induce opioid withdrawal symptoms comprising adverse reactions in central nervous, cardiovascular, gastrointestinal, and respiratory systems (see Table 9.1).

TABLE 9.1. The symptoms of opioid withdrawal.

Body systems affected	Symptoms expressed
Central nervous system	Irritability
	Anxiety
	Restlessness
	Diaphoresis
	Eye watering
	Trembling
	Seizures
Cardiovascular system	Hypertension or hypotension
	Tachycardia
	Ventricular arrhythmias
	Cardiac arrest
Gastrointestinal system	Diarrhea
	Nausea
	Vomiting
Respiratory system	Dyspnea
	Pulmonary edema
	Runny nose
	Sneezing

THE USE OF NALOXONE FOR TREATMENT
OF OPIOID-INDUCED CONSTIPATION

In the case of opioid-dependent individuals maintained on methadone, it is possible to precipitate an acute opioid withdrawal reaction by administering oral naloxone at a dose one-tenth that of the methadone, although considerable variation exists between individuals. Changing the ratio to 5 percent largely eliminates this risk.[13] However, it is apparent that even with the oral use of naloxone, withdrawal is a possibility that must be guarded against.

Accordingly, the first use of naloxone in man to reverse opioid-induced constipation was in an experimental context employing loperamide as the source of gut slowing in order to avoid the possibility of systemic withdrawal.[14] This was a double-blind placebo-controlled trial in which 9 volunteers received 16 mg loperamide alone, 16 mg loperamide with 2 different doses of naloxone by mouth (16 mg and 32 mg), and placebo in random order. Loperamide alone increased the mean transit time, measured by the lactulose hydrogen breath test, by about 30 percent (to 128.8 ± 32.9 minutes, $p < 0.05$) compared with the other three treatments, during which the transit time remained essentially the same (88.8, 84.4, and 85.5 minutes, respectively). Thus, naloxone nullified the gut-slowing effect of loperamide, implying that naloxone could act peripherally to reverse the constipating effects of an opioid.

It was noted that when the glucuronide of naloxone was administered to morphine-dependent rats the result was diarrhea, but little evidence of central opioid withdrawal symptoms was exhibited.[15] This was taken to indicate that naloxone could be delivered to the large bowel by means of the colonic bacterial breakdown of its glucuronide conjugate. However, the findings also suggested that it might be possible to reverse opioid-induced constipation without antagonizing central opioid effects, such as analgesia.

This possibility was supported by further animal work in which intestinal transit time was measured in rats given 1, 2.5, or 5 mg/kg morphine with or without 10 mg/kg naloxone. In addition, the effect of naloxone on analgesia was assessed by measuring the change in hotplate tail-flick latency following administration of 2.5 mg/kg morphine with or without 10 mg/kg naloxone.[16] Naloxone abolished the transit slowing caused by 1 mg/kg morphine, reduced that in response to the 2.5 mg/kg dose by approximately 60 percent ($p < 0.01$) and that in response to the 5 mg/kg dose by approximately 30 percent ($p < 0.05$). Naloxone produced no significant impairment of lengthening of tail-flick latency seen after morphine administration, even though the morphine dose used was less than the maximum given in the transit time part of the study. Interestingly, there was no detectable naloxone in the plasma at the dose level that produced these effects.

Table 9.2 summarizes six clinical studies that have been reported concerning the use of oral naloxone to treat opioid-induced constipation. In addition, a pharmaceutical company (Roxane)-sponsored international multicenter trial was abandoned at a relatively advanced stage and has not been reported as far as the author can ascertain. All reported studies are small.

Study by Culpepper-Morgan et al., 1992

This was an uncontrolled, dose-ranging study performed on three chronic pain patients taking oxycodone with, in two cases, methadone as well.[17] Constipation was not defined specifically, but since starting on opioid analgesics some months before, all the patients had required laxatives in order to be able to defecate. Opioid doses were stable. The purpose of the study was to determine if naloxone by mouth could relieve constipation due to opioids without reducing analgesia.

The initial dose of naloxone was 0.5 mg daily and this was titrated over an undisclosed period to a maximum of 16 mg per day, titration being halted if adequate laxation or significant withdrawal symptoms (assessed on a Himmelsbach scale[18]) occurred. Plasma naloxone levels were assayed in all subjects.

Two subjects were titrated to a naloxone dose of 12 mg daily and experienced spontaneous defecation without adverse effects. The third developed abdominal cramping but without actual defecation even at the 16 mg dose level. However, at this point she also reported symptoms of systemic withdrawal. The peak plasma levels of naloxone in this patient reached 8.0 ng/mL, compared with 6.1 ng/mL and less than 5 ng/mL in the others. In each case levels of naloxone glucuronide were much higher than those of the active drug. It was noted that the time to peak plasma level varied considerably between subjects, possibly reflecting different states of small bowel motility

TABLE 9.2. Clinical studies of oral naloxone for management of opioid-induced constipation.

Authors	Study design	Subject type and number	Opioid type(s) and dose	Naloxone dose	Outcome measures	Results
Culpepper-Morgan et al., 1992	Uncontrolled dose ranging	Chronic pain $n = 3$	Oxycodone 5-60 mg per 24 h, methadone 30-100 mg per 24 h	Initial dose 0.5 mg p.o. once daily, titrated to: Patient A: 12 mg od Patient B: 12 mg bd Patient C: 12 mg od	Spontaneous defecation and symptoms of impending laxation	Patients A and C experienced spontaneous defecation. Patient B had symptoms of abdominal cramps but no defecation; she also had symptoms of opioid withdrawal.
Sykes, 1991 and 1996	Phase I: placebo controlled, double blind	Hospice cancer patients Phase 1: $n = 17$	Oral morphine	Given as a proportion of the morphine dose; Phase 1: 0.5%, 1%, 2%, 5%, 10%, 20%	Phase 1: small bowel transit time, bowel function, adverse effects	Phase 1: no change in transit time. Acute onset of diarrhea in both patients who received naloxone at 20% level. No withdrawal or return of pain.
	Phase 2: uncontrolled, dose ranging	Phase 2: $n = 10$		Phase 2: 10%, 20%, 40%, 80%	Phase 2: transit time omitted	Phase 2: Seven patients experienced laxation. One also had acute withdrawal. One had return of pain without laxation. Overall: Nine out of 12 patients receiving naloxone at 20% or more of the morphine dose experienced laxation.

Latasch et al., 1997	Dose ranging with control period	Unclear. Patients on regular opioids and requiring laxatives. $n = 15$	Morphine	Given as a proportion of the morphine dose: initially 100%, later reducing	Clinical evidence of laxation, withdrawal and adverse effects	Twelve patients experienced a strong and rapid laxative effect. Eleven had a 10-15% loss of analgesia and four experienced withdrawal. Laxative effects were maintained on lower doses of naloxone, representing 2-15% of the naloxone dose.
Meissner et al., 2000	Dose ranging with control period		Morphine in 16 cases, buprenorphine in 1.	Initial dose 3 mg tid, titrating to a maximum of 12 mg tid	Stool frequency, laxative use, pain intensity, adverse effects	Stool frequency = 2.1 (±0.9) without naloxone, 3.5 (±1.4) with naloxone. Laxative use = 6.0 (±0.0) without naloxone, 3.8 (±3.7) with naloxone (all results based on six-day periods). Four patients had significant withdrawal symptoms but none had return of pain.
Hawkes et al., 2001	Single blind, placebo controlled	Healthy volunteers	Codeine 30 mg bid	Naloxone 10 mg bid in an enteric coated sustained release formulation	Whole gut transit time	Gut slowing effects of codeine were offset by naloxone, which also accelerated transit compared with baseline.
Liu and Wittbrodt, 2002	Double blind, randomized controlled trial		Oxycodone 40-120 mg per 24 h in five cases. Morphine 90-1050 mg per 24 h	Three groups: Placebo Naloxone 2 mg tid Naloxone 4 mg tid	Stool frequency, constipation assessment scale, pain intensity, adverse effects	Increase in stool frequency in all patients taking naloxone. Tendency to lower scores on constipation assessment scale. Three patients experienced relapse of pain and withdrawal symptoms.

affecting naloxone absorption. It was also noted that despite the rapid metabolism of naloxone into the glucuronide, there was a dose-dependent increase in plasma area under the curve values. The subject who experienced withdrawal did so not only after a 16 mg naloxone dose but also after two 12 mg doses were given only three hours apart. The study authors proposed that since the terminal elimination half-life of oral naloxone is about two hours, the dosing interval should be at least six hours, on the basis of three times the half-life.

Culpepper-Morgan and co-workers concluded that naloxone by mouth did indeed offer the possibility of therapeutic use as an agent against opioid-induced constipation, but that there was a risk of precipitating unpredictable withdrawal effects in that it depended on both individual variation in absorption and metabolism of naloxone from the gut but also the degree of preexisting tolerance and physical dependence.

Studies by Sykes, 1991 and 1996

This was a two-phase study that was the subject of a preliminary report and then a full account some years later.[19-20] The objective of the study was the same as for the Culpepper-Morgan et al. work just described,[17] but here the population from which subjects were drawn was a group of cancer patients receiving morphine as part of palliative care in a hospice unit. For the first phase a double-blind randomized controlled dose-ranging design was used in which each patient received both naloxone and placebo in random order. The dose of naloxone was linked to the prevailing morphine dose in one of a number of set proportions: naloxone as 0.5 percent, 1 percent, 2 percent, 5 percent, 10 percent, or 20 percent of the quantity of morphine the patient was receiving for pain. All patients required a regular laxative while taking morphine and had no preopioid history of constipation. The primary outcome measures were small bowel transit time assessed by the lactulose hydrogen breath test and pain according to a four-point descriptive scale. Note was made of adverse effects that might represent withdrawal, although no specific scale was used.

The purpose in linking morphine and naloxone doses was to reduce the risk of precipitating the return of pain or the onset of withdrawal symptoms. The reasoning behind it was that in animal work, the slowing effect of morphine on gastrointestinal transit is dose related in a manner that is described by an equation according to the receptor occupation theory of drug response.[21] Similarly, in rodents it had been shown that the antagonism of this action of morphine by naloxone is also dose dependent[22] and appears to rely on competition at a common receptor.[23] It was therefore concluded that the naloxone doses required to provide a laxative effect without reversing analgesia might be proportional to the oral morphine doses causing the constipation, and if the study dosing regime were organized in this way, the risk of adverse effects might be minimized. However, exactly what this proportion should be did not emerge clearly from the literature and hence a dose-ranging approach was adopted.

Two patients were given each of the first 3 dose levels and 4 received the 10 percent level. No change was noted in pain scores, small bowel transit time or adverse effects between placebo and active drugs over this dose range. However, the first two subjects to receive naloxone at 20 percent of their morphine dose experienced a marked laxative effect amounting to diarrhea within as little as 30 minutes. There was no return of pain or occurrence of withdrawal symptoms. Despite this clinical response, small bowel transit time did not change in the patient who consented to complete the assessment. The other subject refused to continue the lactulose hydrogen breath test as he felt the result was apparent clinically. The reason for this surprising lack of apparent effect on small bowel activity may have been the difficulty in standardizing and controlling diet in this patient group, together with the past exposure of some patients to lactulose which may have influenced handling of the marker by intestinal flora. A further problem that became apparent during this phase of the trial was that many patients could distinguish active drug from placebo by the bitter taste of the naloxone.

Accordingly, the second phase of the trial was an open dose-ranging study using the same clinical outcome measures but comparing subjects' stool frequency and consistency, not with their performance on placebo, but with that prior to study entry. Measurement of small bowel transit time was not performed. The progression of naloxone dose as a proportion of morphine dose was now 20 percent, 40 percent, and 80 percent. Ten patients took part in phase two of the study, and seven of these experienced a laxative response, four when taking the 20 percent level and three at higher levels. Thus, combining the two phases of the study, nine out of twelve subjects who took naloxone at 20 percent or more of their morphine dose showed laxation, whereas none of the 14 who took it at the 10 percent level or less had any bowel response.

Adverse effects arose with two patients in the second phase. One had a marked increase in pain (1.5 to 3.0 on a 4-point scale) on moving from the 10 percent to the 20 percent dose level and reported systemic withdrawal symptoms, but there was no laxation. The second had a severe immediate withdrawal reaction, including diarrhea, at the 20 percent dose level, but had no return of pain.

The conclusion of the study was similar to that of Culpepper-Morgan et al.: Naloxone is capable of reversing opioid-induced constipation but with a risk of precipitating pain or withdrawal in susceptible individuals. Also, the laxative response could be undesirably fierce. An attempt was made to draw up guidelines for the experimental therapeutic use of naloxone as a laxative, suggesting a starting point of 20 percent of the morphine dose subject to a maximum initial dose of 5 mg. From this, the concern of subsequent investigators became less the proving of whether naloxone could have a laxative effect in patients taking opioids but rather the selection and titration of doses for safety and efficacy.

Study by Latasch et al., 1997

This study[24] was performed by the same German group that had conducted animal work on naloxone in gut slowing by opioids.[16] It enrolled 15 patients with opioid-related constipation into an open dose-ranging trial using their previous bowel pattern as the control. As the group's studies in rats had found that naloxone could be used orally in doses four times that of the current dose of morphine without reducing analgesic effects, they opted to conduct dose ranging in the opposite direction from Culpepper-Morgan et al.[17] and Sykes.[20] An initial naloxone dose of 100 percent that of morphine was proposed for two days, followed by a reduction to the 50 level on the third and fourth day and then 25 percent on days five and six. Outcome measures were laxative effect, pain visual analog scale scores and withdrawal symptoms.

Twelve of the 15 patients had a strong laxative effect from 1 to 4 hours after commencing naloxone at the 100 percent dose level. Eleven of them had a 10 to 15 percent reduction of analgesia at the same time, which was corrected by a similar increase in morphine dose without restoring constipation. Four had frank symptoms of withdrawal, which responded to a single dose of morphine equivalent to their daily morphine intake. The originally planned regimen of downward naloxone titration was abandoned, and on the second day the naloxone dose was reduced to between 2 and 15 percent of morphine dose. This dose level apparently continued to produce a laxative effect. The failure of naloxone as a laxative in the remaining three patients was attributed to the presence of neurological defects and the effect of concurrent nonopioid drugs.

Thus, the laxative effect of oral naloxone in opioid-taking patients was again confirmed, but the use of very high naloxone doses relative to prevailing morphine doses resulted in an unacceptable degree of adverse effects. Although a relationship between morphine and naloxone doses had been part of the study's original hypothesis, the hasty reduction in naloxone doses following the appearance of side effects made it impossible to tell whether any such relationship actually existed.

Study by Meissner et al., 2000

This was also a prospective case control study in 22 cancer patients who had taken opioid analgesia for at least four weeks and needed laxatives at least 50 percent of the time.[25] A six-day control period on conventional therapy was followed by a period on naloxone, beginning with a four-day titration period from an initial dose of 3 mg t.i.d. to 6 mg t.i.d. on day 2, 9 mg t.i.d. on day 3, and a maximum of 12 mg t.i.d. on day 4 according to laxative and withdrawal response. A further six-day observation period ensued, and the stool frequency and need for laxatives was compared between this and the control period. The Himmelsbach scale[18] was used for assessment of withdrawal symptoms.

Five patients were withdrawn from the study; only one of them experienced withdrawal, clearly as a result of the experimental intervention. The 17 remaining patients took morphine, apart from one, who was maintained on buprenorphine. Fourteen subjects showed a laxation response, usually within two or three days of starting titration, and nine were able to reduce their use of conventional laxatives. In the responding group the stool frequency per six days rose from

2.12 ± 0.9 during the control period to 3.5 ± 1.4 while taking naloxone ($p < 0.01$). Similarly, the days with laxative medication reduced from 6.0 ± 0.0 to 3.8 ± 2.7 (again, $p < 0.01$).

Four patients had Himmelsbach scores between 5 and 12 of a possible 18. In three the symptoms resolved after a modest reduction in naloxone dose, but the fourth patient wished to withdraw from the study. In three cases the naloxone dose was 6 or 9 mg, but the other subject had, in error, received a single dose of 20 mg. Pain scores and mean morphine doses did not vary significantly between control and naloxone periods. One of the patients was followed for over a year, and it was reported that the laxative effect was enduring.

The mean naloxone dose was 17.5 ± 10.2 mg/day, representing 7.5 percent of the mean prevailing morphine dose of 232 mg/day. Of note, there was no significant correlation between morphine dose and effective naloxone dose ($r = -0.38, p = 0.14$).

This study[25] was the first to provide statistical evidence of the effectiveness of oral naloxone as a laxative in constipation caused by morphine. It also cast strong doubt on the theory that naloxone and morphine doses were related. However, despite the trial's careful naloxone dose titration, it still produced troublesome withdrawal symptoms—although not pain—in around 25 percent of the participants. Despite the small size of individual studies and their different design, preventing the combination of results, there had now emerged a clear impression that naloxone did indeed have therapeutic potential in this area. However, it was also a consistent finding that a proportion of patients would suffer opioid withdrawal symptoms, sometimes severely, that would limit the chances of acceptance in clinical practice.

Study by Hawkes et al., 2001

This was a single-blind, controlled trial in 12 healthy male volunteers.[26] Subjects took placebo, codeine, naloxone, or codeine plus naloxone in varied but not randomized order. All preparations were identical in appearance, and when a single active agent was used, a placebo was given as well so that the medication volume remained the same whatever the phase of the trial. Each phase of the trial lasted nine days with a two-week washout period in between. Volunteers were encouraged to maintain a consistent diet throughout. The principal outcome was whole-gut transit time, measured by a radio-opaque marker technique.

Naloxone was used at a dose of 10 mg b.i.d., given in a formulation designed to delay drug release until the terminal ileum, and then provide a sustained release in the colon over the next six hours. A potential advantage of this formulation was to limit the rise in naloxone plasma levels and hence diminish the risk either of return of pain or onset of withdrawal, but this could not be fully tested in the study design.

The trial exposed the variability in individual response to codeine, associated with the CYP2D6 enzyme phenotype. Only eight volunteers showed a gut-slowing response to the 30 mg b.i.d. dose of codeine that was used. However, in this subset codeine lengthened the mean transit time from 50.4 ($\pm$3.0) hours to 66.2 ($\pm$4.2) hours, $p = 0.001$. Naloxone more than offset this increase, giving a transit time of 42.4 ($\pm$5.4) hours when combined with morphine, $p = 0.034$. Interestingly, naloxone also shortened transit time compared with control when used on its own, both in codeine responders and nonresponders: the overall mean of 53.1 ($\pm$3.0) hours in the control period for the whole group fell to 42.1 ($\pm$3.7) hours with naloxone. This finding should be compared with the work of Kreek et al.[27] in idiopathic constipation (reviewed later in this chapter). Some subjects experienced a degree of urgency of defecation, but none had diarrhea.

The study conclusion was that oral naloxone was capable of reversing the gut slowing induced by an opioid, in this case codeine. It was thus supportive of the findings of the clinical studies reviewed previously. The originators of the enteric slow-release formulation of naloxone are clearly hopeful that through its delayed and gradual release of naloxone, it might overcome the difficulties with withdrawal symptoms and return of pain that have been experienced with administration of immediate release preparations. It is said that naloxone plasma levels resulting from the delayed release formulation are considerably lower than those reported by Culpepper-Morgan et al. However, since none of the participants had pain and the opioid was given in low doses of short duration, it was not possible to determine from this study whether the promise of freedom from adverse effects can be fulfilled.

Study by Liu and Wittbrodt, 2002

This study aimed to discover whether, by using low doses of oral naloxone, opioid-induced constipation could be alleviated without precipitating pain or withdrawal.[28] Nine chronic pain patients, some with cancer and some with nonmalignant pain, were randomized to receive placebo, naloxone 2 mg t.i.d., or naloxone 4 mg t.i.d. Each treatment option was therefore taken by only three individuals. All patients dated a history of constipation to the start of their opioid therapy and were on stable analgesic doses. All of them also received conventional laxatives. Outcome measures were stool frequency, the Constipation Assessment Scale,[29] and pain, as measured by the Short Form Brief Pain Inventory.[30] No specific assessment of withdrawal appears to have been made.

In view of the small numbers, no attempt at calculations of statistical significance was made, but the mean stool frequency per week across the assessable members of the group rose from 2.6 prior to the study to 4.4 during it, supporting a clinical impression of improved laxation. However, two patients quickly withdrew from the study, one with complete reversal of analgesia and another with a marked increase in pain. The latter was receiving placebo. The former needed his opioid dose more than doubled to control the pain and did not return to his usual opioid and pain levels for three days after naloxone had been stopped. Interestingly, he was taking the highest dose of opioid of any participant in the trial (Oxycodone extended release 40 mg b.i.d. and 80 mg qhs, plus 20 mg oxycodone prn).

In three cases a substantial increase in opioid dose was necessary: 42 percent and 50 percent in two subjects, each of whom was receiving naloxone 2 mg t.i.d., and 67 percent in a patient on placebo. Again, the patients on naloxone required their increased opioid dose for several days, whereas the one who had been on placebo recovered her original pain levels as soon as the study medication was stopped.

Liu and Wittbrodt concluded, similar to Meissner's group,[25] that there was no relationship between the laxative dose of naloxone and that of morphine. Indeed, they noted that in their very small sample those most sensitive to naloxone in terms of suffering adverse effects tended to be on the highest opioid doses. In terms of absolute doses, 2 mg t.i.d. was adequate for some patients. However, they write, "Due to the significant risk of decreasing analgesic efficacy of the opioids, a better agent would be an opioid antagonist that does not cross the blood-brain barrier."

Multicenter Trial by Roxane Laboratories, Inc.

This international multicenter placebo-controlled trial is understood to have recruited significantly in the United States and in continental Europe before being terminated because of "lack of efficacy." Enquiry by the author has failed to elicit details of the therapeutic failure of naloxone, and he has not traced any report of the results of the trial prior to abandonment. It may be that a larger and more rigorously conducted study than any of those detailed here showed, as so often the case, that the benefits of a drug claimed by reports of smaller, poorly controlled trials were exaggerated. However, on the basis of the uniform conclusion of the trials that have been published—that naloxone can produce laxation in opioid-induced constipation, sometimes all too powerfully—it seems surprising if no such effect was found. It would be more understandable if the trial had confirmed what has also been a universal finding of these preliminary studies—that naloxone is prone to cause withdrawal symptoms or return of pain in an unpredictable way, which may make it impossible for it to gain a license for this use.

DISCUSSION OF REPORTED CLINICAL STUDIES

Two common themes emerge from these small trials, none of which can be given a Jadad quality score of more than 3 out of 5.[31] The first is that oral naloxone will often produce clinical laxation in patients experiencing constipation as a result of opioid analgesia. This laxation is liable to be rapid in onset and may be diarrheal in severity.

The second theme is that even by mouth, naloxone can cause either opioid withdrawal symptoms or can impair the analgesic efficacy of opioids. Strategies that have been adopted to control this risk have been either to use low starting doses of naloxone (Culpepper-Morgan et al.[17] and Liu and Wittbrodt[28]) or to link the naloxone dose to the patient's opioid dose (Sykes[20]) or, potentially, a combination of these.

The dose linkage strategy has been invalidated. What was over-looked in the definition of this strategy was that the studies which informed it had been conducted on animals, and that those animals had a brief or fairly brief history of opioid exposure. The evidence from human studies of those with long-term use of opioids is that the reaction to opioid antagonists is proportional not to the opioid dose but to the degree of opioid tolerance.[32] Thus, in direct opposition to the assumptions of the strategy, patients on the highest opioid doses might need the *smallest* doses of naloxone. The results of at least three of the studies (Culpepper-Morgan et al.,[17] Sykes,[20] and Liu and Wittbrodt[28]) are consistent with this possibility, in that the most severe adverse reactions tended to be in subjects taking above-average opioid doses.

The solution to this problem might be to start with a low dose of naloxone. But, if so, how low? Sykes recommended individual starting doses no higher than 5 mg, on the basis that the withdrawal reactions which had been observed had occurred after individual naloxone doses of 7 mg and 20 mg. Culpepper-Morgan's group found that their patient who had such reactions did so after naloxone 12 mg to 16 mg, but warned that too frequent dosing might, through accumulation, result in withdrawal at doses lower than this. Meissner et al. discovered withdrawal after doses as low as 6 mg, while Liu and Wittbrodt found significant reversal of analgesia in some patients after doses as low as 2 mg. These symptoms are unpleasant, a fact rendered all the more important by the considerations, first, that constipation is not a life-threatening complaint and, second, that the target for this use of naloxone is patients who are receiving analgesia in order to improve their quality of life.

The questions must be asked whether opioid antagonists can provide an oral treatment for opioid-induced constipation and, if so, whether naloxone is the appropriate member of this class of drug to use. Except for the unreported Roxane study, naloxone has shown evidence of improving bowel function when opioids are being taken. However, it seems inappropriate to use a medication for symptomatic relief that carries at least a 15 percent risk of undoing the pain control that has been achieved or of adding potentially distressing adverse effects of its own.

An enteric release formulation of naloxone has been tested in a healthy volunteer group taking codeine, but not to date in patients requiring opioid pain relief and who have taken opioids for substantial periods of time.[32] These conditions are the real test of this use of an opioid antagonist. Enteric release might smooth the body's exposure to naloxone and make it less likely that glucuronidation mechanisms would be overcome and result in increased circulating levels of the active drug. However, it remains a fact that there is bound to be variability in the ability of individuals both to conjugate naloxone and then to break down that glucuronide back into active naloxone. More important, it is clear that the ability to tolerate circulating naloxone without experiencing withdrawal or reversal of analgesia is highly variable and difficult to foresee. One cannot "convert" from a morphine dose to a balancing dose of naloxone, but would need a careful titration process from a very low initial dose (perhaps, as in Culpepper-Morgan et al.'s work, 0.5 mg). The lines of defense are limited, because once naloxone has entered circulation, it will penetrate the CNS relatively easily. A greater margin of security would be offered by an antagonist that is both poorly absorbed from the intestine and enters the CNS from the circulation only with difficulty. Quaternary opioid antagonists, such as methylnaltrexone and alvimopan (see Chapters 10 and 11), appear to fulfil these criteria and therefore to offer potentially more fruitful lines of research for the future than can naloxone.

USE OF ORAL NALOXONE FOR IDIOPATHIC CONSTIPATION

Endogenous opioids have a physiological but not fully clarified role in the control of gut function (see Chapters 1 and 2). It is therefore possible that in some cases of idiopathic bowel conditions producing constipation, there is a relative overactivity of endogenous opioid systems. Hence, the reduction of the effects of such activity by an opioid antagonist might be therapeutic. This hypothesis has been tested in four studies, two of which are by Hawkes' group, one of these having been discussed previously. Both other reports are from Kreek and colleagues at the Rockefeller University in New York.

Study by Kreek, Schaefer, et al., 1983

The first Kreek report consists of case studies of two women with long-standing chronic constipation requiring daily oral laxatives with addition of enemas and suppositories.[27] Initially both patients were given an intravenous infusion of naloxone. They then received oral naloxone 3.6 mg six times a day (a total of 21.6 mg per 24 hours) in a single-blind fashion, one of them crossing over to a placebo preparation. It is not clear whether these interventions were deemed to constitute a formal trial. The outcome measures were fecal wet and dry weights. Both women showed a marked increase in fecal weights while taking naloxone, although statistics were not appropriate. One of them had her first spontaneous bowel action without the use of suppositories or enemas in over a year.

Study by Kreek, Paris, et al., 1983

The second Kreek report, made only in abstract form, concerned 25 elderly people not taking opioid medications but with a regular need for laxative interventions.[33] After a one week baseline assessment period, subjects were given naloxone 8 mg t.i.d. or placebo in what was described as a double-blind random crossover design for four weeks. Stools were collected for wet weight estimations and the stool frequency noted. Missing data resulted in the exclusion of five participants. Of the remainder, 13 showed a significant ($p < 0.05$) increase in stool weight while taking naloxone compared with the placebo phase. Five people complained of adverse effects when they were receiving naloxone, namely indigestion (two individuals), gas pain, dizziness, and abdominal pain. However, 14 complained of a variety of symptoms while taking placebo.

From both reports the authors concluded that naloxone by mouth produced improvement in bowel function in a proportion of cases of idiopathic constipation, suggesting that in these responding individuals, endogenous opioids played a role in producing the gut slowing.

Study by Hawkes et al., 2002

Hawkes et al. reported a randomized, double-blind, placebo-controlled trial of naloxone in irritable bowel syndrome (IBS) patients with constipation.[34] The same enteric sustained release form of naloxone was used as in their previous study, delivering 10 mg naloxone twice daily. Following a two-week baseline period, patients received either naloxone or placebo for eight weeks. Bowel function and IBS symptoms were recorded, together with details of the bowel function and laxative use.

Twenty-eight patients entered the trial, 22 of them female. One withdrew from the naloxone group because of nausea and vomiting; two were lost from the placebo group owing to noncompliance. There was a trend toward greater improvement in IBS symptoms with naloxone than with placebo, but there was no change in stool frequency or consistency with either treatment. Quality-of-life scores across a range of domains also tended to improve more with naloxone than with placebo. The trial was suggestive rather than statistically conclusive, but the suggestion was in favor of naloxone.

DISCUSSION OF REPORTED STUDIES OF NALOXONE FOR IDIOPATHIC CONSTIPATION

There is limited evidence stemming from a very small number of trials, none involving large numbers of patients, that oral naloxone can have a therapeutic effect in a proportion of individuals with idiopathic constipation. How clinically significant such effects are and what categories of patients can benefit from naloxone remain to be determined. Nonetheless, this is a potentially exciting new treatment avenue for individuals who may experience persistent discomfort from their bowel dysfunction. This clinical area may also be more appropriate for the further evaluation of naloxone than that of opioid-induced constipation, as there is no risk of precipitating pain or withdrawal symptoms. For the same reason, there is no evident reason to suppose that quaternary opioid antagonists would have any advantage over naloxone, and so it may be here that this drug finds its niche in gastroenterology.

NOTES

1. Gan TJ, Ginsberg B, Glass PSA, Fortney J, Jhaveri R, Perno R. Opioid-sparing effects of a low-dose infusion of naloxone in patient-administered morphine sulfate. *Anesthesiology* 1997;87:1075-1081.

2. Margolin S. Decreased gastrointestinal propulsive activity after intracranial morphine. *Fed Proc* 1954;13:383-384.

3. Green AF. Comparative effects of analgesics on pain threshold, respiratory frequency and gastrointestinal propulsion. *Br J Pharmacol* 1959;14:26-34.

4. Manara l, Bianchetti A. The central and peripheral influences of opioids on gastrointestinal propulsion. *Annu Rev Pharmacol Toxicol* 1985;25:249-273.

5. Porreca F, Mosberg HI, Hurst R, Hruby VJ, Burks TF. Roles of mu, delta and kappa opioid receptors in spinal and supraspinal mediation of gastrointestinal transit effects and hot-plate analgesia in the mouse. *J Pharmacol Exp Ther* 1984;230: 341-348.

6. Manara L, Bianchi G, Ferretti P, Monferini E, Strada D, Tavani A. Local and CNS-mediated effects of morphine and narcotic antagonists on gastrointestinal propulsion in rats. In Leong Way E (ed). *Endogenous and exogenous opiate agonists and antagonists.* New York: Pergamon; 1980:143-146.

7. Manara L, Bianchi G, Ferretti P, Tavani A. Inhibition of gastrointestinal transiti by morphine in rats results primarily from direct drug action on gut opioid sites. *J Pharmacol Exp Ther* 1986;237:945-948.

8. Daniel EE, Sutherland WH, Gogoch A. Effects of morphine and other drugs on motility of the terminal ileum. *Gastroenterology* 1959;36:510-523.

9. Ruppin H. Review: Loperamide—A potent antidiarrhoeal drug with actions along the alimentary tract. *Aliment Pharmacol Ther* 1987;1:179-190.

10. Zaks A. Jones T, Fink M, Freedman AM. Naloxone treatment of opiate dependence. *JAMA* 1971;215:2108-2110.

11. Fishman J, Roffwarg H, Hellman L. Disposition of naloxone-7, 8-^{3}H in normal and narcotic-dependent men. *J Pharmacol Exp Ther* 1973;187:575-580.

12. Albeck H, Woodfield S, Kreek MJ. Quantitative and pharmacokinetic analysis of naloxone in plasma using high performance liquid chromatography with electrochemical detection and solid-phase extraction. *J Chromatogr* 1989;488:435-445.

13. Kreek MJ, Gutjahr CL, Garfield JW, Bowen DV, Field FH. Drug interactions with methadone. *Ann N Y Acad Sci* 1976;281:350-370.

14. Basilisco G, Camboni G, Bozzani A, Paravicini M, Bianchi PA. Oral naloxone antagonizes loperamide-induced delay of orocaecal transit. *Dig Dis Sci* 1987;32:829-832.

15. Simpkins JW, Smulkowski M, Dixon R, Tuttle R. Evidence for the delivery of narcotic antagonists to the colon as their glucuronide conjugates. *J Pharmacol Exp Ther* 1988;244:195-205.

16. Jurna I, Kaiser R, Kretz O, Baldauf J. Oral naloxone reduces costipation but not antinociception from oral morphine in the rat. *Neurosci Lett* 1992;142:62-64.

17. Culpepper-Morgan JA, Inturrisi CE, Portenoy RK et al. (1992) Treatment of opioid-induced constipation with oral naloxone: A pilot study. *Clin Pharmacol Ther* 1992;52:90-95.

18. Himmelsbach CK. The morphine abstinence syndrome, its nature and treatment. *Ann Intern Med* 1941;15:829-839.

19. Sykes NP. Oral naloxone in opioid-associated constipation. *Lancet* 1991;337: 1475.

20. Sykes NP. An investigation of the ability of oral naloxone to correct opioidrelated constipation in patients with advanced cancer. *Palliat Med* 1996;10:135-144.

21. Bianchi G, Feretti P, Recchia M, Rocchetti M, Tavani A, Manara L. Morphine tissue levels and reduction of gastrointestinal transit in rats. *Gastroenterology* 1983;85:852-858.

22. Wong C-L, Roberts MB, Wai M-K. Effect of morphine and naloxone on intestinal transit in mice. *Eur J Pharmacol* 1980;64:289-295.

23. Parolaro D, Sala M, Gori E Effect of intracerebroventricular administration of morphine upon intestinal motility in rats and its antagonism with naloxone. *Eur J Pharmacol* 1977;46:329-338.

24. Latasch L, Zimmerman M, Eberhardt B, Jurna I. Treatment of morphine-induced constipation with oral naloxone [German]. *Anaesthesist* 1997;46:191-194.

25. Meissner W, Schmidt U, Hartmann M, Kath R, Reinhart K. Oral naloxone reverses opioid-associated constipation. *Pain* 2000;84:105-109.

26. Hawkes ND, Richardson C, Evans BK, Rhodes J, Lewis SJ, Thomas GA. Effect of an enteric-release formulation of naloxone on intestinal transit in volunteers taking codeine. *Aliment Pharmacol Ther* 2001;15:625-630.

27. Kreek MJ, Schaefer RA, Hahn EF, Fishman J. Naloxone, a specific opioid anatagonist, reverses chronic idiopathic constipation. *Lancet* 1983;1:261-262.

28. Liu M, Wittbrodt E. Low-dose oral naloxone reverses opioid-induced constipation and analgesia. *J Pain Symptom Manage* 2002;23:48-53.

29. McMillan SC, Williams FA. Validity and reliability of the Constipation Assessment Scale. *Cancer Nurs* 1989;12:183-188.

30. Cleeland CS, Ryan KM. Pain assessment: Global use of the Brief Pain Inventory. *Ann Acad Med Singapore* 1994;23:129-138.

31. Jadad A. *Randomised Controlled Trials. 1998.* London: BMJ Publishing Group; 1998.

32. Wikler A, Fraser HF, Isbell H. N-allylnormorphine: Effects of single doses and precipitation of acute abstinence syndromes during addiction to morphine, methadone or heroin in man. *J Pharmacol Exp Ther* 1953;109:8-20.

33. Kreek MJ, Paris P, Bartol MA, Mueller D. Effects of short term administration of the specific opioid antagonist naloxone of fecal evacuation in geriatric patients. *Gastroenterology* 1983;86:1144.

34. Hawkes ND, Rhodes J, Evans BK, Rhodes P, Hawthorne AB, Thomas GA. Naloxone treatment for irritable bowel syndrome—A randomized controlled trial with an oral formulation. *Aliment Pharmacol Ther* 2002;16:1649-1654.

Chapter 10

Methylnaltrexone: Investigations in Treating Opioid Bowel Dysfunction

Thomas A. Boyd
Chun-Su Yuan

Opioid compounds, which are widely administered for a variety of medical indications, are associated with a number of side effects, especially opioid bowel dysfunction. Opioid-induced bowel dysfunction, often described as constipation, is found in 90 percent of patients treated with opioids[1] and is a significant problem in 40 to 45 percent of patients with advanced cancer.[2-4] Very often, opioid constipation is severe enough to limit opioid use and prevents achievement of the adequate dose used for pain therapy.[4-6] Although this clinical problem has a significant negative impact on the quality of life of these patients, the issue has received insufficient attention in the past from the medical community.[7]

Naltrexone (see Figure 10.1A) is a clinically prescribed opioid antagonist. Like other tertiary opioid receptor antagonists, such as

This work is supported in part by National Institutes of Health grant R01 CA79042, and grant M01 RR00055 from the U.S. Public Health Service General Clinical Research Center.

Methylnaltrexone was originally formulated and subsequently modified by faculty at the University of Chicago. It is currently being developed by Progenics Pharmaceuticals, Inc. Dr. Boyd is an employee of Progenics Pharmaceuticals, Inc. The University of Chicago and Dr. Yuan stand to benefit financially from the further development of methylnaltrexone.

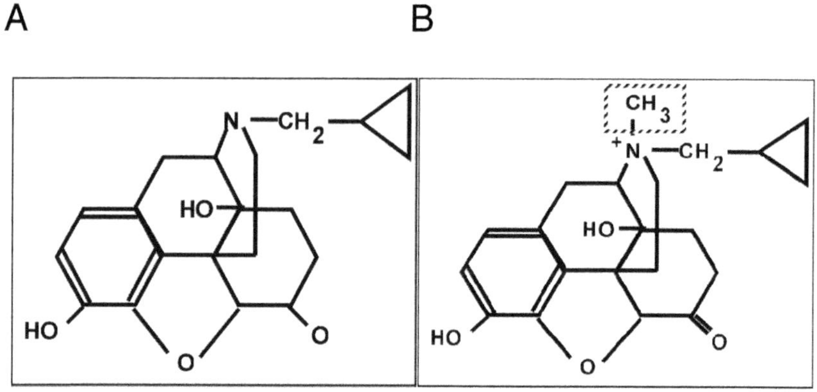

A   B

FIGURE 10.1. Chemical structures of (A) naltrexone and (B) methylnaltrexone.

naloxone and nalmefene, it is fairly lipid soluble and readily crosses the blood-brain barrier. Thus, these drugs block both the beneficial pain-relieving and the adverse effects of opioids. Selective antagonism of opioid gut side effects by tertiary compounds with specific dose regimens has been attempted. Success, however, has been limited by the propensity for these antagonists to reverse analgesia or to induce opioid withdrawal.[8-13]

Methylnaltrexone or *N*-methylnaltrexone bromide (Figure 10.1B) is a unique peripheral opioid receptor antagonist currently under clinical investigation.[14] Methylnaltrexone is a quaternary derivative of naltrexone.[15] The addition of the methyl group at the ring amine of naltrexone forms methylnaltrexone, a compound with greater polarity and lower lipid solubility. Due to these properties, methylnaltrexone does not cross the blood-brain barrier in humans.[15,16] Methylnaltrexone offers the therapeutic potential to reverse the undesired side effects of opioids that are mediated by receptors located in the periphery (e.g., in the gastrointestinal tract) without affecting analgesia or precipitating opioid withdrawal symptoms that are predominantly mediated by receptors in the central nervous system.

Methylnaltrexone is a white, odorless powder that is freely soluble in water. Methylnaltrexone has been formulated for clinical trials as a sterile solution for injection or infusion and as a solid to be administered orally in capsules or tablets.

RECEPTOR-BINDING STUDIES

Methylnaltrexone antagonizes opioid binding at μ opioid receptors (IC_{50} of 70 nM). It has a relatively lower affinity for κ opioid receptors (IC_{50} of 575 nM), and it does not interact with δ opioid or orphanin receptors. It also does not bind significantly to any nonopioid receptors. In addition, methylnaltrexone has no intrinsic opioid agonist activity as measured in standard pharmacological models of analgesia, gastrointestinal motility, or in behavioral tests designed to detect substitutes for narcotics.[17-19] Thus, methylnaltrexone would be categorized as a pure antagonist.

In the gastrointestinal tract, methylnaltrexone exhibits selectivity for μ receptors. This was demonstrated in isolated gastric-brainstem preparations from neonatal rats. In this preparation, opioid agonists produce a marked, dose-dependent decrease in brainstem neuronal firing when the drugs are applied solely to the gastric compartment.[20] Methylnaltrexone antagonized the inhibitory effects of morphine and those of the μ-selective opioid agonist, DAMGO (*trans*-3,4-dichloro-*N*-methyl-*N*[2-(1-pyrrolidinyl)cyclohexyl]benzeneacetamide methanesulfonate hydrate) in a competitive manner, with 50 percent inhibition observed at approximately 300 nM. Methylnaltrexone was 18.8-fold less potent as an antagonist of the κ-selective agonist, U-50,488H, and it was ineffective against the δ-selective agonist, DPDPE (D-Pen[2], D-Pen[5]-enkaphalin).[21]

PRECLINICAL STUDIES

Morphine and other opioids produce a slowing of normal gut function.[22] When methylnaltrexone was administered subcutaneously to rats, it antagonized the delaying effects of morphine on the transit time of a charcoal meal through the gut.[18] Methylnaltrexone at doses of 1, 3, or 10 mg/kg were effective in a dose-dependent manner when given 15 minutes prior to morphine (see Figure 10.2). Methylnaltrexone did not affect morphine analgesia when administered subcutaneously, although it did reduce analgesia when given intracerebroventricularly. These findings not only illustrate the ability of methylnaltrexone to reverse the gut-slowing action of morphine but also suggest that it does not enter the central nervous system in phar-

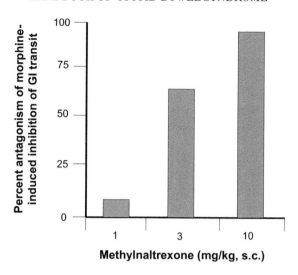

FIGURE 10.2. Inhibition by methylnaltrexone of morphine-induced slowing of gastrointestinal transit in rats. *Source:* Adapted from Gmerek DE, Cowan A, Woods JH. Independent central and peripheral mediation of morphine-induced inhibition of gastrointestinal transit in rats. *J Pharmacol Exp Ther* 1986;236:8-13. Reprinted with permission.

macologically significant amounts. Similar findings have been reported by other laboratories.[23] Methylnaltrexone can act directly on the gastrointestinal tract. For example, it prevented the inhibition by morphine of electrically induced contractions in isolated guinea pig ileum.[24] Further, in isolated smooth muscle strips from guinea pig ilea and human small intestine, methylnaltrexone produced concentration-dependent antagonism of morphine-induced inhibition of electrically stimulated contractions.[25] Interestingly, in the human small intestine preparation, methylnaltrexone by itself enhanced the force of muscle contraction by about 30 percent.[25] This suggests the presence of a background level of endogenous opioid activity in the gut tissue and opens the possibility of employing methylnaltrexone as a therapeutic agent in situtations where endogenous opioids in the periphery contribute to human pathology.

Emesis is common side effect of opioid therapy. Dogs are highly susceptible to morphine-induced emesis and have been used as a model of this side effect. In a study conducted in dogs, methylnaltrexone pretreatment by either the intramuscular or intravenous route produced dose-related antagonism of the emetic effects of morphine.[26] The emetic effect of the opioid was completely blocked at a methylnaltrexone dose of 0.25 mg/kg i.m. or 0.2 mg/kg i.v. ($p < 0.05$) (see Figure 10.3). In another study, the combined administration of methylnaltrexone (0.25 mg/kg i.v.) plus morphine (1 mg/kg) reduced both apomorphine- and cisplatin-induced emesis in dogs.[27] In this study, it was hypothesized that morphine may have both peripheral emetic effects and central antiemetic effects, and the combination of methylnaltrexone plus morphine unmasked a centrally mediated antiemetic activity of morphine.

Recently, using a rat model of simulated emesis (increase kaolin intake), we evaluated whether methylnaltrexone decreases morphine-induced kaolin consumption. We observed that after morphine, kaolin intake increased significantly compared to intake in the vehicle group, and the increase could be attenuated by ondansetron administration. Methylnaltrexone dose-dependently reduced kaolin ingestion induced by morphine.[28]

Control of the cough reflex is thought to reside in the central nervous system, but peripheral mechanisms might be important. In a

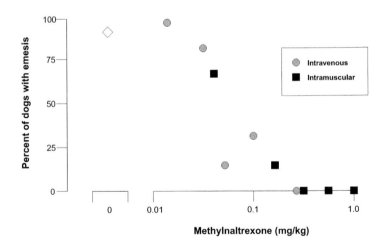

FIGURE 10.3. Inhibition by methylnaltrexone of morphine-induced emesis in dogs. *Source:* Adapted from Foss JF, Bass AS, Goldberg LI. Dose-related antagonism of the emetic effect of morphine by methylnaltrexone in dogs. *J Clin Pharmacol* 1993;33:747-751.

study conducted in guinea pigs, it was shown that methylnaltrexone (2.0 mg/kg i.p.) blocked the suppression of cough due to morphine injection.[29] This dose had no effect on antinociception due to morphine. Naltrexone, which is capable of entering the brain, antagonized cough suppression but also reversed morphine-induced analgesia at doses as low as 0.16 mg/kg i.p. This study suggests that peripheral receptors play a role in cough control, and that methylnaltrexone may have benefit as an agent to maintain the cough reflex in patients receiving opioids.

The opioid antagonism of methylnaltrexone is dose dependent and reversible. In gastrointestinal transit studies in rats, methylnaltrexone's antiopioid activity becomes attenuated as time elapses between the administration of methylnaltrexone and the administration of the opioid.[18,23] Similarly, the antiemetic effect in morphine-treated dogs decreases over the period between 60 and 180 minutes after dosing.[26] In a study in dogs where methylnaltrexone was shown to inhibit morphine-induced spike potentials in duodenal smooth muscle (the electrical signal correlates with circular smooth muscle contraction characteristic of the interdigestive state),[16] subcutaneous doses of 5 mg/kg methylnaltrexone produced an effect that could be measured as long as 50 minutes after dosing, whereas the effects of lower doses could not be measured beyond 25 minutes postdosing. These findings suggest that methylnaltrexone's opioid antagonist activity is reversible at the level of the receptors and that the magntitude of its pharmacologic action will be dependent on the local concentration of the drug at the receptor sites in the tissue.

The literature notes instances in rodents in which high doses of methylnaltrexone were associated with antinociception, suggesting a possible central effect.[23] The partial reversal of analgesia at high doses in rodents may be indicative of metabolic conversion of methylnaltrexone to naltrexone in rodents, which is known to occur at a low rate in these species.[30] This type of conversion is also low in dogs and appears to be very low in humans.[30] In keeping with its inability to cross the blood-brain barrier, systemically administered methylnaltrexone, in contrast to tertiary opioid antagonists, is not associated with the precipitation of withdrawal in animals or humans that have been treated with opioids. In acutely opioid-dependent dogs, methylnaltrexone (1 to 50 mg/kg s.c.) did not produce behavioral signs of withdrawal,[16] nor did it precipitate clinical signs of withdrawal in opioid-dependent rhesus monkeys.[17,31] When administered intravenously to methadone-treated human subjects at doses that produced laxation, methylnaltrexone did not produce withdrawal symptoms, as determined by means of the employment of recognized scales for assessment of such symptoms.[32]

Methylnaltrexone is also not expected to modify opioid ingestion in habituated subjects. In a rat model of heroin self-administration, methylnaltrexone (30 mg/kg i.p.) did not alter the rate of opioid self-administration.[33]

Animals tolerate doses of methylnaltrexone that are well above the proposed effective range in humans.[16,32] Formal animal toxicology studies are currently being conducted to support the clinical testing program in man.

ABSORPTION, ELIMINATION, AND METABOLISM

The disposition of methylnaltrexone has been studied in animals and, to a limited extent, in humans. Methylnaltrexone concentrations in serum, plasma, or urine can be quantitated using solid-phase extraction and reverse-phase high performance liquid chromatography (HPLC) with electrochemical detection.[34,35] Recently, a newer liquid chromatography/mass spectoscopy/mass spectorscopy (LC/MS/MS) method has been validated and employed to support future development studies (unpublished data).

Methylnaltrexone is readily bioavailable after subcutaneous, intravenous, or oral administration. Plasma concentrations in normal human subjects after s.c. doses of 0.1 or 0.3 mg/kg are proportional to dose. The maximal levels of drug achieved after either a 0.1 mg/kg or a 0.3 mg/kg dose exceed the concentrations required for effective antagonism of opioid binding at receptor sites. The plasma half-life of methylnaltrexone in humans after parenteral administration has been reported variously in the literature to range between 1.5 and 3 hours.[36] The terminal half-life of methylnaltrexone might be several hours longer than this, because the sampling times employed in the early, published studies often did not extend longer than six hours after dosing. More recent investigations suggest that the terminal half-life of the drug in humans might be closer to six to nine hours after parenteral dosing (unpublished data).

Methylnaltrexone is absorbed from the gastrointestinal tract after oral ingestion.[37] Peak plasma levels are much lower than after subcutanous administration of drug. However, with adjustment of the oral dose, similar AUC values can be achieved.[37] Since methylnaltrexone is a charged molecule, gut absorption might be less than complete. Evidence of variability between individuals has been noted. Enterically coated dosage forms have been studied in early clinical trials. The bioavailability of enterically coated methylnaltrexone at oral doses of 3.2 mg/kg and 6.4 mg/kg has been evaluated in normal volunteers.[38] These doses were effective in reducing morphine-induced delays in oral-cecal transit time to levels similar to baseline. There was no correlation of plasma levels of methylnaltrexone with clinical effects in these studies, though. The drug may exert part of its action through direct lumenal action on the intestinal wall. Low doses of enterically coated methylnaltrexone may have clinical utility in treating opioid-induced gastrointestinal immotility.

Elimination of parenterally administered methylnaltrexone has been studied in humans and animals. In humans, the amount of unchanged compound detected in urine over the period of 0 to 6 hours after a subcutaneous dose was 52 percent and 47 percent for doses of 0.1 or 0.3 mg/kg, respectively.[36] A similar fraction was excreted in the urine after intravenous dosing to humans.[30,39,40] A large fraction of parenterally administered drug appears to be eliminated in the feces. In dogs, for example, samples of urine and feces were collected over a period of 120 hours after an intravenous dose of 2 mg ^{14}C-labeled methylnaltrexone. Cumulative recovered radioactivity amounted to 51 percent in urine and 32 percent in feces, the bulk of which was excreted within 24 hours of dosing.[30]

In studies conducted to date, metabolism of methylnaltrexone did not appear to play a major role in its elimination. Drug detected in urine and feces appears to be largely unchanged. Demethylation of methylnaltrexone at the quaternary nitrogen position is of interest, as it would produce naltrexone, which can enter the central nervous system. Demethylation of methylnaltrexone was determined in mice, rats, and dogs administered ^{14}C-labeled methylnaltrexone.[30] N-[^{14}CH$_3$]-methylnaltrexone was prepared by the reaction of [^{14}C]-iodomethane with naltrexone, and a product having a radiochemical purity greater than 99 percent was prepared. Mice and rats were administered single subcutaneous doses of N-[^{14}CH$_3$]-methylnaltrexone

(10 mg/kg) and placed in metabolism cages for collection of expired carbon dioxide. Similarly, beagle dogs fitted with plastic face masks were administered single subcutaneous doses, and expired carbon dioxide was collected. The cumulative percentage of the administered dose excreted as ^{14}C-labeled carbon dioxide over a in two-hour period was 1.17 ± 0.06 percent in rats, 0.48 ± 0.01 percent in mice, and 0.14 ± 0.01 percent in dogs. Disposition of radiolabeled methylnaltrexone was also determined in five patients with metastatic cancer. In four of the five patients, no ^{14}C-labeled carbon dioxide was detectable in breath samples collected at intervals up to 240 minutes postdose. In one patient, the peak rate of activity, determined 15 minutes postdose, was measurable but extremely low (< 0.0001 percent of dose/h), and expired radioactivity was no longer detected at one hour after treatment. Approximately 39 to 53 percent of the dose appeared in the urine within 24 hours of dosing.[30] These studies indicate that although there may be a very low rate of demethylation occurring in rodent species, demethylation is not a pathway of methylnaltrexone metabolism in humans.

SAFETY AND TOLERANCE STUDIES IN HUMANS

In a Phase 1 safety and tolerance study in health volunteers, intravenous methylnaltrexone doses of up to 0.32 mg/kg were given without any side effects. Transient orthostatic hypotension (plasma levels in excess of 1,400 ng/mL) was observed in some subjects after doses of 0.64 to 1.25 mg/kg.[40] This orthostatic hypotension appears unlikely to occur at therapeutic dose levels, since the projected therapeutic dose will be below 0.45 mg/kg. Safety and tolerance data have been obtained in other studies at the University of Chicago in more than 200 subjects who received intravenous methylnaltrexone at doses ranging from 0.3 to 0.45 mg/kg. No significant subjective or objective side effects have been observed.

It was noted previously that humans do not show evidence of demethylation of methylnaltrexone. In another study of opioid effects on the hypoxic drive to breathe, ten healthy volunteers were maintained at a normal end tidal CO_2 while progressive hypoxia was allowed to hemoglobin oxygen saturation of 80 percent. Morphine depressed the normal increases in spontaneous minute ventilation. Intravenous methylnaltrexone 0.3 mg/kg did not reverse the morphine-induced respiratory depression, further demonstrating that the compound does not penetrate into the brain.[41]

Recently, safety and tolerability following repeated intravenous methylnaltrexone administration were evaluated in 12 normal subjects. During the 72-hour study, subjects received 0.3 mg/kg intravenous methylnaltrexone every six hours. No significant adverse effects or changes in vital signs occurred. Maximum concentrations of methylnaltrexone, determined two minutes postdose, were 538 ± 237 (mean ± S.D.) and 675 ± 180 ng/mL after the first and twelfth doses, respectively. Based on a comparison of the areas under the plasma concentration curve (AUC) values after the first and twelfth doses, no clinically significant accumulation of drug was observed.[42]

EFFICACY STUDIES

Efficacy of Parenteral Methylnaltrexone in Normal Subjects

The ability of methylnaltrexone to counteract the gut-inhibitory effects of opioids has been demonstrated in a number of studies. In a study of 12 healthy volunteers, intravenous morphine of 0.05 to 0.1 mg/kg was observed to delay oral-cecal transit time using the lactulose hydrogen breath test.[43,44] This delay of the gut transit time was effectively prevented by a single injection of intravenous methylnaltrexone 0.45 mg/kg.[39] All subjects responded to both the opioid and the peripheral antagonist. Oral-cecal transit time increased after morphine administration in all 12 subjects, and methylnaltrexone prevented morphine-induced delay in every subject (see Figure 10.4). Morphine significantly increased oral-cecal transit time from a baseline of 104.6 ± 31.1 min to 163.3 ± 39.8 min ($p < 0.01$). In contrast, transit time in subjects given methylnaltrexone plus morphine (106.3 ± 39.8 min) was not significantly different from baseline. The compound thus prevented 97 percent of morphine-induced changes in oral-cecal transit time ($p < 0.01$ compared to morphine alone). Using the cold-pressor test,[45] this study also demonstrated that methylnaltrexone does not reverse morphine-induced analgesia.[39]

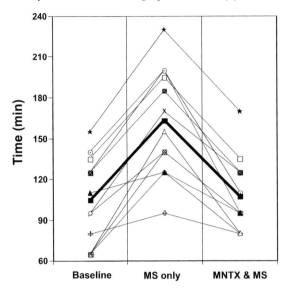

FIGURE 10.4. The individual oral-cecal transit time (ordinate) of 12 healthy volunteers according to the injections (abscissa). The heavy line represents the mean. MS = intravenous morphine (0.05 mg/kg). MNTX = intravenous methylnaltrexone (0.45 mg/kg). *Source:* Reprinted from *Clinical Pharmacology & Therapeutics,* 59, Yuan CS, Foss JF, O'Connor M, Toledano A, Roizen MF, Moss J, Methylnaltrexone prevents morphine-induced delay in oral-cecal transit time without affecting analgesia: A double-blind randomized placebo-controlled trial, 469-475, Copyright 1996, with permission from the American Society for Clinical Pharmacology and Therapeutics.

Morphine, even at low doses, can delay gastric emptying in humans.[46] Murphy et al. conducted a randomized, controlled trial to evaluate the effects of intravenous methylnaltrexone on the opioid-induced delay in gastric emptying.[47] In their study, 11 healthy volunteers were given placebo, morphine, or 0.3 mg/kg methylnaltrexone plus morphine on three separate occasions. The rate of gastric emptying was measured by a noninvasive epigastric bioimpedance technique and the acetaminophen absorption test. They observed that the time taken for the gastric volume to decrease to 50 percent ($t_{0.5}$) following ingestion of a fluid load after administration of the placebo was 5.5 ± 2.1 min (mean $\pm$ SD). Morphine prolonged the gastric emptying $t_{0.5}$ to 21 ± 9.0 min ($p < 0.05$). Methylnaltrexone injection reversed the morphine-induced delay in gastric emptying to a $t_{0.5}$ of 7.4 ± 3.0 ($p < 0.05$). In addition, the maximum concentrations of serum acetaminophen and acetaminophen AUCs from 0 to 90 min after morphine were significantly different from either placebo or morphine administered concomitantly with methylnaltrexone ($p < 0.05$). No difference in maximum acetaminophen concentration or AUCs was noted between placebo and methylnaltrexone plus morphine, indicating a normalization of gastric emptying by methylnaltrexone administration.

Compared to intravenous injection, subcutaneous administration is a more convenient route of delivery medication. In another controlled trial, the efficacy of subcutanous methylnaltrexone in antagonizing the morphine-induced delay in oral-cecal transit time was evaluated in 12 normal subjects. In the first group ($n = 6$), morphine (0.05 mg/kg i.v.) increased the transit time from baseline level of 85 ± 20.5 min to 155 ± 27.9 min ($p < 0.01$). When 0.1 mg/kg methylnaltrexone was administered subcutaneously at the same time as morphine, the transit time was reduced to 110 ± 41.0 min. In the second group ($n = 6$), morphine increased the transit time from a baseline level of 98 ± 49.1 min to 140 ± 58.2 min ($p < 0.01$). After subcutaneous methylnaltrexone (0.3 mg/kg) plus morphine, the transit time was reduced to 108 ± 59.6 min ($p < 0.05$). Pharmacokinetic data showed that the time to peak plasma concentration was approximately 20 min.[36] These data suggest that subcutaneous methylnaltrexone may have clinical utility in treating opioid-induced gut side effects.

Efficacy of Oral Methylnaltrexone in Normal Subjects

Early clinical studies have indicated that oral methylnaltrexone is safe and well tolerated in humans. In a study of 14 normal, healthy subjects, no adverse effects were observed after single oral doses of methylnaltrexone at levels up to 19.2 mg/kg.[37] Oral-cecal transit time was also measured in that study in the presence and absence of coadministered intravenous morphine. The results showed that the delay of the oral-cecal transit time after morphine was effectively prevented by the oral medication with methylnaltrexone in a manner proportional to the dose of the antagonist (see Figure 10.5).

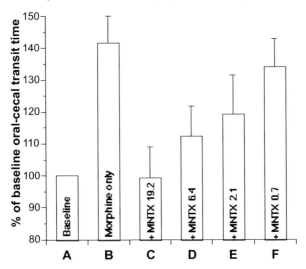

FIGURE 10.5. Dose-related response of oral methylnaltrexone of oral-cecal transit time in 14 healthy volunteers. Placebo plus placebo (A) is normalized to 100%. Placebo plus intravenous morphine 0.05 mg/kg (B) significantly increases the transit time. Intravenous morphine (0.05 mg/kg) was administered 20 min after oral methylnaltrexone in C, D, E, and F. Oral methylnaltrexone 19.2 mg/kg plus intravenous morphine 0.05 mg/kg (C) completely prevents morphine-induced increase in the transit time. Oral-cecal transit time changes after the lower methylnaltrexone doses of 6.4, 2.1, 0.7 mg/kg plus intravenous morphine 0.05 mg/kg are shown in D, E, and F, respectively. MNTX = oral methylnaltrexone (mg/kg). *Source:* Reprinted from *Clinical Pharmacology & Therapeutics,* 61, Yuan CS, Foss JF, Osinski J, Toledano A, Roizen MF, Moss J. The safety and efficacy of oral methylnaltrexone in preventing morphine-induced delay in oral-cecal transit time, 467-475, Copyright 1997, with permission from the American Society for Clinical Pharmacology and Therapeutics.

In that study,[37] the investigators also observed a rapid initial increase in plasma levels within 5 to 20 min after administration of regular, or uncoated, compound, suggesting a correlation to gastric drug absorption. Because changes in gastric emptying time do not affect constipation significantly, we hypothesized that the delivery of relatively higher amounts of methylnaltrexone to the bowel would exert a more direct, possibly lumenal effect on the intestine. Subsequently, we conducted another double-blind, randomized, placebo-controlled study to evaluate the efficacy of orally administered, enteric-coated methylnaltrexone. The coating prevented degradation or release of the drug in the stomach but allowed release in the small and large intestine. This prevented gastric absorption and achieved lower plasma levels of the compound. In the study,[38] it was observed that gut transit time was prolonged after morphine administration in our subjects, and that a low dose of enteric-coated methylnaltrexone (3.2 mg/kg) completely prevented the morphine-induced increases in oral-cecal transit time. Plasma concentrations after enteric-coated methylnaltrexone 6.4 mg/kg and 3.2 mg/kg were substantially lower compared to those after administration of the uncoated formulation. These results suggest that there might be a prevailing direct or local effect of enteric-coated methylnaltrexone, and that the enteric-coated formulation may exert pharmacological actions on the gut more efficiently on a milligram per kilogram basis.

Efficacy of Methylnaltrexone in Chronic Opioid Users

In a study of 19 methadone-maintained, opioid-dependent volunteers, 58 percent of subjects reported constipation. The oral-cecal transit time of these methadone-maintained individuals was 159 ± 49.2 min, which was significantly longer than the transit time recorded in our previous normal human volunteer studies ($p < 0.01$). The results indicated that tolerance to opioids does not appear to extend to gastrointestinal motility and transit. Subjects on chronic methadone therapy are therefore a good model in which to evaluate the gut effects of opioid antagonists.[48] These subjects could be used as a proxy group for advanced cancer patients with chronic opioid-induced constipation.

A pilot study was then conducted to evaluate the effects of methylnaltrexone in four chronic methadone subjects with constipation (daily methadone dose: 38 to 90 mg/kg).[49] All of these subjects had immediate laxation responses during and after intravenous medication (0.05 to 0.45 mg/kg). Gut transit times were reduced significantly from the baseline levels. At the highest dose (0.45 mg/kg), one subject experienced severe abdominal cramping but showed no other signs of systematic withdrawal such as lacrimation, diaphoresis, mydriasis, or hallucinations. It appears that chronic opioid users are more sensitive to opioid antagonists compared to the opioid-naive subjects recruited in our previous trials.

A subsequent double-blind, randomized, placebo-controlled trial enrolled 22 chronic methadone subjects (daily methadone dose: 30 to 100 mg) with opioid-induced constipation.[32] For this two-day study with daily intravenous methylnaltrexone (0.1 ± 0.1 mg/kg) administrations, the effects on observed bowel movement (laxation), oral-cecal transit time, and central opioid withdrawal symptoms were determined. The 11 subjects in the placebo group showed no laxation response; the 11 subjects in the methylnaltrexone group had an immediate laxation response after intravenous methylnaltrexone ($p <$ 0.01). Most subjects reported mild to moderate abdominal cramping after methylnaltrexone, which they described as being similar to a defecation sensation without significant discomfort. Bowel movements, in most cases, were loose and large in quantity. As shown in Figure 10.6, baseline (predose) oral-cecal transit times for subjects in the methylnaltrexone and placebo groups averaged a little over two hours (132.3 and 126.8 min, respectively). The average change in the methylnaltrexone-treated group after treatment with the drug was a decrease of 77.7 ± 37.2 min. This was significantly greater than the average change in the placebo group (-1.4 ± 12.0 min) ($p < 0.01$). There was no opioid withdrawal observed in either group, and no significant side effects were reported by the subjects during the study. The data suggested that patients receiving chronic opioids also may have increased sensitivity to methylnaltrexone, and low dose methylnaltrexone may have a potential clinical utility in managing opioid-induced constipation.

Based on a case report, methylnaltrexone was successfully treated a 70-year-old palliative care patient with end-stage cryptogenic cirrhosis and fentanyl-patch-induced intractable constipation. Intravenous methylnaltrexone (0.3 to 0.4 mg/kg per day) induced laxation without affecting analgesia. No significant adverse effects were observed.[50]

Due to the fact that oral administration is a more convenient way to deliver the drug to some subjects, the efficacy of oral methylnaltrexone on 12 methadone-maintained subjects was also investigated.[51] None of the subjects showed a laxation response to placebo on day 1. On day 2, after receiving 0.3 mg/kg methylnaltrexone, three out of four subjects had a bowel movement, with the time between drug administration and laxation averaging 18.0 ± 8.7 hr. Higher doses of methylnaltrexone were associated with a reduced time to laxation.

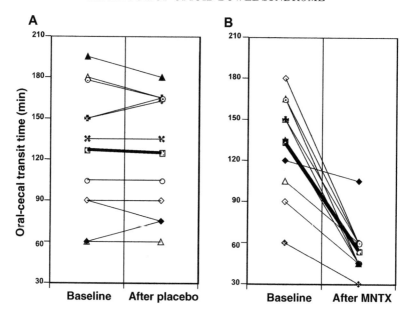

FIGURE 10.6. Changes in individual oral-cecal transit time of chronic metha-done subjects. (A) The transit time (ordinate) of 11 subjects in the placebo group from baseline to after placebo injection (abscissa). (B) The transit time (ordinate) of 11 methadone subjects in methylnaltrexone (MNTX) group from baseline to after study drug administration (abscissa). The heavy line represents the mean. The average change in the methylnaltrexone group was significantly greater than the average change in the placebo group ($p < 0.001$). *Source:* Adapted from Yuan CS, Foss JF, O'Connor M, Osinski J, Karrison T, Moss J, Roizen MF. Methylnaltrexone for reversal of constipation due to chronic methadone use: A randomized controlled trial. *JAMA* 2000;283:367-372.

All subjects in 1.0 mg/kg group ($n = 4$) and 3.0 mg/kg group ($n = 4$) had bowel movements at 12.3 ± 8.7 and 5.2 ± 4.5 h after receiving the oral compound, respectively. Oral methylnaltrexone had a significant dose-response effect ($p < 0.05$), while plasma drug levels were very low or undetectable. No opioid withdrawal occurred in any subjects, and no adverse effects were reported.

Recently, Thomas et al. reported results from a Phase 2 double-blind, randomized, parallel group, dose-ranging study of subcutane-ous methylnaltrexone in subjects with advanced medical illness and symptomatic opioid-induced constipation despite the use of laxatives.[52] Patients were on stable opioid therapy and had constipation for at least 48 hours at study entry. Subjects were randomized to 1 of 4 doses of methylnaltrexone (1, 5, 12.5, or 20 mg) and treated in a double-blinded fashion every other day for one week. Laxation within 4 or 24 hours of dosing, symptoms of withdrawal, pain, and side effects were monitored after each dose. Following this double-blind period, subjects could continue on methylnaltrexone in an open-label protocol, with an allowance for titration of the dose to optimize the laxation effect over a three-week period. Approximately one-half to two-thirds of patients laxated within four hours of receiving a dose of methylnaltrexone of 5 mg or higher during the double-blind period, as compared with 11 percent of subjects at the 1 mg dose. The response rate within 24 hours escalated to between 57 and 72 percent at the higher doses as compared with approximately 31 percent at the 1 mg dose. The percent of patients who laxated within four hours of each double-blind dose is presented in Figure 10.7. The proportion of patients with laxation responses within four hours of dosing after ad-

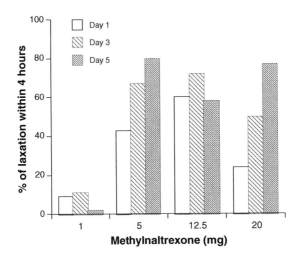

FIGURE 10.7. Methylnaltrexone produced laxation responses in subjects with chronic opioid-induced constipation. Thirty-three hospice patients were administered one of four randomized doses of subcutaneous methylnaltrexone (1, 5, 12.5, or 20 mg) on a blinded basis every other day for three doses. Laxation responses within four hours of methylnaltrexone dosing were determined. Methylnaltrexone statistically significantly increased four-hour laxation rates in subjects administered 5 mg or greater, *p* < 0.0001, versus the 1 mg group.

ministration of 5 mg or more was tested against that in the 1 mg dose group, using a Fisher's exact test. The *p* value for all doses ≥ 5 mg combined compared with 1 mg was < 0.0001. Figure 10.8 illustrates reports of laxation on treatment days and no-treatment days in the double-blind period. The number and percent of subjects with laxation on no-treatment days was lower than on treated days for all dose groups, and was markedly lower for the patients who received methylnaltrexone doses of 5 mg or higher. Thus, for those patients who received doses of 5 mg or higher, laxation occurred predominantly on days when they received methylnaltrexone.

In addition, patients who received methylnaltrexone doses of 5 mg or higher usually experienced laxation within a few minutes to a few hours after dosing. Figure 10.9 shows Kaplan-Meier plots for the dosing groups. The median time to laxation after methylnaltrexone doses of 5 mg or greater was approximately one hour. The frequency of laxation also increased. The subjects reported median values of two or fewer bowel movements in the week prior to double-blind dosing. After double-blind treatment, the median number of laxations per week increased to 2.3 in the 1 mg group and to 3.5 to 5.8 at methylnaltrexone doses of 5 mg and higher (see Figure 10.10).

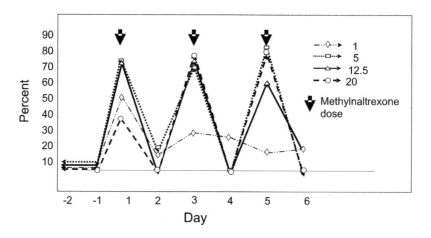

FIGURE 10.8. Laxation responses in methylnaltrexone-treated hospice patients on dosing and nondosing days. The number and percent of subjects with laxation within 24 hours of dosing on treatment days was higher than on non-treatment days in all dose groups ($p < 0.01$), and was markedly higher in subjects who received methylnaltrexone doses of 5 mg or higher.

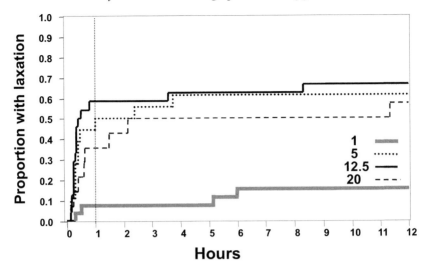

FIGURE 10.9. Kaplan-Meier plots of time to laxation (in hours) in hospice subjects after administration of 1, 5, 12.5, or 20 mg methylnaltrexone. The log rank test indicated $p < .0001$.

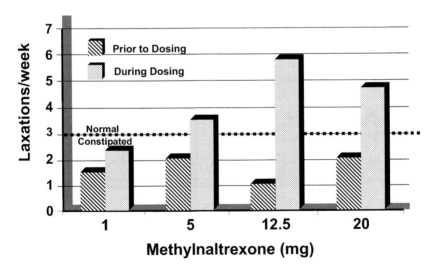

FIGURE 10.10. Methylnaltrexone at doses of 5 mg or higher increased the median number of laxations per week in hospice subjects during the double-blind phase of dosing.

The laxation responses were also examined with respect to methylnaltrexone dose in milligrams per kilogram. The laxation responses within four hours of dosing for all double-blind doses, with doses expressed in mg/kg, is presented in Figure 10.11. It shows similar results to those shown for fixed milligram doses. The lowest dose group roughly corresponds to the 1 mg dose level. Again, the responses of the two higher dose groups were not different from each other.

During the open-label phase, the median dose level administered was 7.5 mg. Laxations appear to be dose related. Within 4 hours of dosing, the percent of subjects with laxation were 49 percent, 60 percent, 63 percent, 50 percent, and 100 percent with methylnaltrexone doses of 5, 7.5, 10, 12.5, and 15 mg, respectively (see Figure 10.12). The results within 24 hours of dosing were similar.

Withdrawal or increased pain was not observed. The most common side effects were abdominal cramping and flatulence, but all were transient. The data suggest that methylnaltrexone is well tolerated in the hospice population and that it produces a dose-related laxation effect in up to 70 percent of patients within 4 hours of dosing.

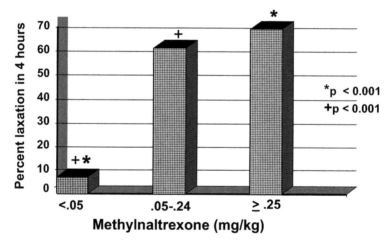

FIGURE 10.11. Laxation responses in relation to methylnaltrexone administration during the double-blind phase of dosing in hospice subjects, expressed on a milligram per kilogram basis. Methylnaltrexone doses in the ranges of 0.05 to 0.25 mg/kg and >0.25 mg/kg were associated with a statistically significant increases in rates of laxation within 4 hours of dosing compared with doses <0.05 mg/kg ($p < 0.001$, Fisher's exact test).

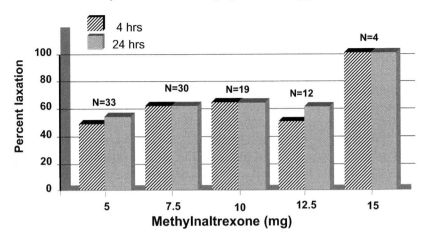

FIGURE 10.12. Laxation associated with methylnaltrexone administration during the open-label phase of the study in hospice subjects. Following the conclusion of the double-blind dosing phase, all subjects entering the open-label phase were started on 5 mg methylnaltrexone, after which titration of the dose was permitted.

SUMMARY

As the first peripheral opioid receptor antagonist, methylnaltrexone provides us with an opportunity to elucidate the mechanism of the peripheral effects of opioids, especially in humans. Among the potential applications of methylnaltrexone,[14,53] the prevention and treatment of opioid-induced gut adverse effects has been studied most to date. At present, many patients receiving opioid pain medications must choose between burdensome side effects or ineffective analgesia. Based on the data presented in this chapter, the clinical utility of methylnaltrexone in preventing or treating opioid-induced constipation is promising. The completion of large-scale clinical trails is warranted; it appears that methylnaltrexone has the potential to alleviate opioid side effects in patients with pain while allowing continued use of opioid analgesics.

Editor's Note

Since completion of this chapter, Progenics Pharmaceuticals, Inc. (www.progenics.com) has completed the following clinical studies on methylnaltrexone.

In March 2005, Progenics reported positive results from a multi-center, double-blind, placebo-controlled, Phase 3 clinical trial of methylnaltrexone for the treatment of opioid-induced constipation in 154 patients with advanced medical illness. The primary endpoint of the trial was whether a single subcutaneous dose of methylnaltrexone induced laxation within four hours. The results showed that a single dose of methylnaltrexone at 0.15 mg/kg or 0.30 mg/kg induced laxation within four hours at more than four times the rate of placebo. On average, laxation occurred within about one hour in the methyl-naltrexone-treated patients. These results were highly statistically significant, and the drug was generally well tolerated. A second trial involving repeated dosing of methylnaltrexone or placebo in this group of patients is ongoing.

In addition, early 2005, Progenics reported positive results from a multi-center, double-blind, placebo-controlled, Phase 2 clinical trial of methylnaltrexone for the management of post-operative bowel dysfunction in 65 patients. Patients who received intravenous doses of 0.3 mg/kg methylnaltrexone following major abdominal surgery exhibited an acceleration of gastrointestinal recovery by at least one day on average compared to placebo. Significant improvements were seen in clinically important measures of gastrointestinal recovery: time to first bowel movement and discharge eligibility from the hospital. Methylnaltrexone was generally well tolerated, with no reports of serious adverse events related to the drug.

NOTES

1. Twycross RG, Lack SA. *Symptom control in far advanced cancer: Pain relief.* London: Pitman;1983.

2. Walsh TD. Oral morphine in chronic cancer pain. *Pain* 1984;18:1-11.

3. Cameron JC. Constipation related to narcotic therapy: A protocol for nurses and patients. *Cancer Nurs* 992;15:372-377.

4. Glare P, Lickiss JN. Unrecognized constipation in patients with advanced cancer: A recipe for therapeutic disaster. *J Pain Symptom Manage* 1992;7:369-371.

5. Portenoy RK. Constipation in the cancer patient: Causes and management. *Med Clin North Am* 1987;71:303-311.

6. McCaffrey M, Beebe A. Managing your patients' adverse reactions to narcotics. *Nursing* 1989;19:166-168.

7. Meier DE, Morrison RS, Cassel CK. Improving palliative care. *Ann Intern Med* 1997;127:225-230.

8. Gowan JD, Hurtig JB, Fraser RA, Torbicki E, Kitts J. Naloxone infusion after prophylactic epidural morphine: Effects on incidence of postoperative side-effects and quality of analgesia. *Can J Anaesth* 1988;35:143-148.

9. Jaffe JH, Martin WR. Opioid analgesics and antagonists. In Gilman AG, Rall TW, Nies AS, Taylor P (eds.), *The pharmacological basis of therapeutics.* New York: Pergamon Press; 1990:485-521.

10. Sykes NP. Oral naloxone in opioid-associated constipation. *Lancet* 1991; 337:1475.

11. Cheskin LJ, Chami TN, Johnson RE, Jaffe JH. Assessment of nalmefene glucuronide as a selective gut opioid antagonist. *Drug Alcohol Depend* 1995; 39:151-154.

12. Culpepper-Morgan JA, Inturrisi CE, Portenoy RK, Foley K, Houde RW, Marsh F, Kreek MJ. Treatment of opioid-induced constipation with oral naloxone: A pilot study. *Clin Pharmacol Ther* 1992;52:90-95.

13. Sykes NP. Using oral naloxone in management of opioid bowel dysfunction. In Yuan CS (ed.), *Handbook of Opioid Bowel Syndrome.* Binghamton, NY: The Haworth Press; 2005;175-195.

14. Yuan CS, Foss JF. Methylnaltrexone: Investigation of clinical applications. *Drug Dev Res* 2000; 50:133-141.

15. Brown DR, Goldberg LI. The use of quaternary narcotic antagonists in opiate research. *Neuropharmacology* 1985;24:181-191.

16. Russell J, Bass P, Goldberg LI, Schuster CR, Merz H. Antagonism of gut, but not central effects of morphine with quaternary narcotic antagonists. *Eur J Pharmacol* 1982;78:255-261.

17. Woods JH, Medzihradsky F, Smith CB, Young AM, Swain HH. Annual report: evaluation of new compounds for opioid activity (1980). *NIDA Res Monogr* 1981;34:327-366.

18. Gmerek DE, Cowan A, Woods JH. Independent central and peripheral mediation of morphine-induced inhibition of gastrointestinal transit in rats. *J Pharmacol Exp Ther* 1986;236:8-13.

19. Walker MJ, Le AD, Poulos CX, Cappell H. Role of central versus peripheral opioid receptors in analgesia induced by repeated administration of opioid antagonists. *Psychopharmacology (Berl)* 1991;104:164-166.

20. Yuan CS. Gastric effects of mu-, delta- and kappa-opioid receptor agonists on brainstem unitary responses in the neonatal rat. *Eur J Pharmacol* 1996;314:27-32.

21. Yuan CS, Foss JF. Gastric effects of methylnaltrexone on mu, kappa, and delta opioid agonists induced brainstem unitary responses. *Neuropharmacology* 1999;38:425-432.

22. Manara L, Bianchetti A. The central and peripheral influences of opioids on gastrointestinal propulsion. *Annu Rev Pharmacol Toxicol* 1985;25:249-273.

23. Bianchi G, Fiocchi R, Tavani A, Manara L. Quaternary narcotic antagonists' relative ability to prevent antinociception and gastrointestinal transit inhibition in

morphine-treated rats as an index of peripheral selectivity. *Life Sci* 1982;30:1875-1883.

24. Valentino RJ, Herling S, Woods JH, Medzihradsky F, Merz H. Quaternary naltrexone: Evidence for the central mediation of discriminative stimulus effects of narcotic agonists and antagonists. *J Pharmacol Exp Ther* 1981;217:652-659.

25. Yuan CS, Foss JF, Moss J. Effects of methylnaltrexone on morphine-induced inhibition of contraction in isolated guinea-pig ileum and human intestine. *Eur J Pharmacol* 1995;276:107-111.

26. Foss JF, Bass AS, Goldberg LI. Dose-related antagonism of the emetic effect of morphine by methylnaltrexone in dogs. *J Clin Pharmacol* 1993;33:747-751.

27. Foss JF, Yuan CS, Roizen MF, Goldberg LI. Prevention of apomorphine- or cisplatin-induced emesis in the dog by a combination of methylnaltrexone and morphine. *Cancer Chemother Pharmacol* 1998;42:287-291.

28. Aung HH, Mehendale SR, Xie JT, Moss J, Yuan CS. Methylnaltrexone prevents morphine-induced kaolin intake in the rat. *Life Sci* 2004;74:2685-2691.

29. Foss JF, Orelind E, Goldberg LI. Effects of methylnaltrexone on morphine-induced cough suppression in guinea pigs. *Life Sci* 1996;59:PL235-PL238.

30. Kotake AN, Kuwahara SK, Burton E, McCoy CE, Goldberg LI. Variations in demethylation of N-methylnaltrexone in mice, rats, dogs, and humans. *Xenobiotica* 1989;19:1247-1254.

31. Valentino RJ, Katz JL, Medzihradsky F, Woods JH. Receptor binding, antagonist, and withdrawal precipitating properties of opiate antagonists. *Life Sci* 1983; 32:2887-2896.

32. Yuan CS, Foss JF, O'Connor M, Osinski J, Karrison T, Moss J, Roizen MF. Methylnaltrexone for reversal of constipation due to chronic methadone use: A randomized controlled trial. *JAMA* 2000;283:367-372.

33. Koob GF, Pettit HO, Ettenberg A, Bloom FE. Effects of opiate antagonists and their quaternary derivatives on heroin self-administration in the rat. *J Pharmacol Exp Ther* 1984;229:481-486.

34. Kim C, Cheng R, Corrigall WA, Coen KM. High-perfomance liquid-chromatography with Coulometric Electochemical detection. *Chromatographia* 1989;28:359-363.

35. Osinski J, Wang A, Wu JA, Foss JF, Yuan CS. Determination of methylnaltrexone in clinical samples by solid-phase extraction and high-performance liquid chromatography for a pharmacokinetics study. *J Chromatogr B Analyt Technol Biomed Life Sci* 2002;780:251-259.

36. Yuan CS, Wei G, Foss JF, O'Connor M, Karrison T, Osinski J. Effects of subcutaneous methylnaltrexone on morphine-induced peripherally mediated side effects: A double-blind randomized placebo-controlled trial. *J Pharmacol Exp Ther* 2002;300:118-123.

37. Yuan CS, Foss JF, Osinski J, Toledano A, Roizen MF, Moss J. The safety and efficacy of oral methylnaltrexone in preventing morphine-induced delay in oral-cecal transit time. *Clin Pharmacol Ther* 1997;61:467-475.

38. Yuan CS, Foss JF, O'Connor M, Karrison T, Osinski J, Roizen MF, Moss J. Effects of enteric-coated methylnaltrexone in preventing opioid-induced delay in oral-cecal transit time. *Clin Pharmacol Ther* 2000;67:398-404.

39. Yuan CS, Foss JF, O'Connor M, Toledano A, Roizen MF, Moss J. Methylnaltrexone prevents morphine-induced delay in oral-cecal transit time without af-

fecting analgesia: A double-blind randomized placebo-controlled trial. *Clin Pharmacol Ther* 1996;59:469-475.

40. Foss JF, O'Connor MF, Yuan CS, Murphy M, Moss J, Roizen MF. Safety and tolerance of methylnaltrexone in healthy humans: A randomized, placebo-controlled, intravenous, ascending-dose, pharmacokinetic study. *J Clin Pharmacol* 1997;37:25-30.

41. Amin HM, Sopchak AM, Foss JF, Esposito BF, Roizen MF, Camporesi EM. Efficacy of methylnaltrexone versus naloxone for reversal of morphine-induced depression of hypoxic ventilatory response. *Anesth Analg* 1994;78:701-705.

42. Yuan CS, Doshan H, O'Connor M, Maleckar S.A., Israel R, Moss J. Methylnaltrexone reduces oral-cecal transit time in. *Dig Dis Week* 2003:A824.

43. Bond JH, Jr., Levitt MD, Prentiss R. Investigation of small bowel transit time in man utilizing pulmonary hydrogen (H2) measurements. *J Lab Clin Med* 1975; 85:546-555.

44. Read NW, Al-Janabi MN, Bates TE, Holgate AM, Cann PA, Kinsman RI, McFarlane A, Brown C. Interpretation of the breath hydrogen profile obtained after ingesting a solid meal containing unabsorbable carbohydrate. *Gut* 1985;26:834-842.

45. Yuan CS, Karrison T, Wu JA, Lowell TK, Lynch JP, Foss JF. Dose-related effects of oral acetaminophen on cold-induced pain: A double-blind, randomized, placebo-controlled trial. *Clin Pharmacol Ther* 1998;63:379-383.

46. Yuan CS, Foss JF, O'Connor M, Roizen MF, Moss J. Effects of low-dose morphine on gastric emptying in healthy volunteers. *J Clin Pharmacol* 1998; 38:1017-1020.

47. Murphy DB, Sutton JA, Prescott LF, Murphy MB. Opioid-induced delay in gastric emptying: a peripheral mechanism in humans. *Anesthesiology* 1997;87:765-770.

48. Yuan CS, Foss JF, O'Connor M, Moss J, Roizen MF. Gut motility and transit changes in patients receiving long-term methadone maintenance. *J Clin Pharmacol* 1998;38:931-935.

49. Yuan CS, Foss JF, O'Connor M, Osinski J, Roizen MF, Moss J. Effects of intravenous methylnaltrexone on opioid-induced gut motility and transit time changes in subjects receiving chronic methadone therapy: A pilot study. *Pain* 1999;83:631-635.

50. Yuan CS, Moss J, Wei G, Maleckar SA, Boyd TA, Israel RJ. Methylnaltrexone for chronic opioid-induced constipation. *Proc Am Soc Clin Oncol* 2002; 21:376a.

51. Yuan CS, Foss JF. Oral methylnaltrexone for opioid-induced constipation. *JAMA* 2000;284:1383-1384.

52. Thomas J, Portenoy RK, Moehl M, Von Gunten C, Thielemann P, Stambler N, Tran D, Galasso F, Israel R. A phase II randomized dose-finding trail of methylnaltrexone for the relief of opioid-induced constipation in hospice patients. *Proc Am Soc Clin Oncol* 2003;22:2933.

53. Ho WZ, Guo CJ, Yuan CS, Douglas SD, Moss J. Methylnaltrexone antagonizes opioid-mediated enhancement of HIV infection of human blood mononuclear phagocytes. *J Pharmacol Exp Ther* 2003;307:1158-1162.

Chapter 11

Management of Opioid-Induced Bowel Dysfunction and Postoperative Ileus: Potential Role of Alvimopan

Joseph F. Foss
William K. Schmidt

INTRODUCTION

The pharmacologic effects of opioids in the gastrointestinal (GI) tract include inhibition of gastric and intestinal motility, impaired defecation, and increased fluid absorption from the bowel.[1] These symptoms have been attributed to several mechanisms involving both peripheral and central opioid receptors. Opioid receptors have been localized throughout the GI tract,[2,3] and stimulation of these receptors by exogenous opioids has been shown to directly affect bowel function.[4,5] Of the three most prominent opioid receptor subtypes— mu, kappa, and delta—the mu opioid receptor is the primary target for pain management among most currently marketed opioid analgesics;[6] these opioids maintain selectivity for the mu opioid receptor at

The following scientists, clinicians, and principal investigators provided key data in support of this chapter: Randall Carpenter, MD; David Jackson, MD; Bruce Wallin, MD; Wei Du, PhD; Yuju Ma, MS; Mahmoud Seyedsadr, PhD; Deanne Garver, PhD; Lee Techner, DPM; Maryann Cherubini, MFT; Kathie Gabriel, RN (Adolor Corporation, Exton, PA); Andrea Kurz, MD; James Fleshman Jr, MD; Akiko Taguchi, MD; Neeru Sharma, MD (Washington University, St. Louis, MO); H. Randolph Bailey, MD (University of Texas Affiliated Hospitals, Houston, TX); Conor Delaney, MD, PhD (Cleveland Clinic, Cleveland, OH); James Weese, MD (University of Medicine and Dentistry of New Jersey, Newark, NJ); Neil Hyman, MD (Fletcher Allen Health Care, Burlington, VT); Bruce Wolff, MD (Mayo Clinic, Rochester, MN); Fabrizio Michelassi, MD (University of Chicago, Chicago, IL); Todd Gerkin, MD (Central Carolina normal therapeutic doses.[6] However, the mu opioid receptor also appears to be the primary mediator of decreased GI motility, thus causing a potential clinical trade-off between effective analgesia and management of adverse side effects.[6]

Opioid-Induced Bowel Dysfunction (OBD)

Opioid analgesics are efficacious for management of moderate-to-severe chronic pain, but they can have severe and occasionally dose-limiting adverse effects, especially on the GI tract. Although commonly referred to by its most debilitating symptom, constipation, OBD more accurately represents a constellation of multiple GI effects, including abdominal pain and discomfort, bloating, and gastroesophageal reflux. These symptoms are caused by alterations in acetylcholine release at the level of the myenteric and submucosal plexi and alterations in secretion and water absorption from the bowel. Unmanaged OBD can have further consequences, such as nausea and vomiting, fecal impaction, and impaired absorption of drugs.[7] It has been estimated that 33 percent of people in the United States on chronic opioid therapy (including cancer patients, patients with chronic nonmalignant pain, and those receiving methadone for opioid addiction) are affected by opioid bowel dysfunction.[8]

Evidence suggests that peripheral opioid receptors may play a more predominant role in the development of OBD.[1,4,9] In contrast to the peripheral opioid receptors, central opioid receptors appear to play a minor role in the pathogenesis of OBD.[10] Studies in rats show that inhibition of GI motility by systemic morphine results primarily from direct action on gut opioid sites.[11]

Surgery, PA, Greensboro, NC); Daniel Paulson, MD; Daniel Kennedy, PharmD (Veterans Affairs Medical Center, Richmond, VA); William Barr, PharmD, PhD (Medical College of Virginia, Richmond, VA); Spencer Liu, MD (Virginia Mason Medical Center, Seattle, WA); James Fricke, DDS (PPD Development, Austin, TX); Richard Rauck, MD (Bowman Gray School of Medicine, Wake Forest University, Winston-Salem, NC); Joseph Liberto, MD (University of Maryland, College Park, MD); Roger Donovick, MD; Walter Ling, MD (Matrix Institute and UCLA, Los Angeles, CA); Louis Cantilena Jr, MD, PhD (Uniformed Services University of the Health Sciences, Bethesda, MD); John Callaghan, MD (Eli Lilly and Company, Indianapolis, IN); and members of the Alvimopan Postoperative Ileus Study Group and the Alvimopan Opioid Bowel Dysfunction Study Group.

Postoperative Ileus (POI)

Postoperative ileus is a transient impairment of the GI motility following abdominal or other surgery characterized by abdominal distension, lack of bowel sounds, accumulation of gas and fluids in the bowel, and delayed passage of flatus and stool.[12-15] Whereas some of the symptoms of POI are similar to those of OBD (including abdominal distention, lack of bowel sounds, gas and fluid accumulation in the bowel, delayed passage of flatus, and impaired defecation), the etiology of POI is thought to result from a combination of surgical stress, inflammation, sympathetic stimulation, release of inhibitory humoral agents, operative trauma secondary to physical manipulation or transection of the bowel during surgery, anatomical location of surgery, changes in electrolyte and fluid balance, and changes in normal physiologic processes as a result of the use of opioids, inhalation anesthetics, and other drugs used during and following surgery.[16-21] Postoperative ileus may result in added pain and discomfort following surgery, delayed enteral feedings with concomitant potential for compromised nutrition, impaired absorption of orally administered drugs, increased postoperative nausea and vomiting, and delayed mobilization and recovery, all of which may increase patient morbidity, lengthen hospital stays, and increase health care costs.[17-20]

One of the primary mechanisms of POI appears to involve inhibition of neural signaling within the sympathetic nervous system. Of particular importance is the efferent sympathetic reflex that inhibits motility in the intestinal tract.[17,20,21] Endogenous opioid peptides released as a result of surgical insult, as well as exogenous opioids used postoperatively for pain management, can affect intestinal nerve activity.[13-15,22-26] Inhibition of the enteric nervous system and the efferent spinal nerves affects GI motility by interfering with the coordinated propulsive muscle contractions that constitute peristalsis. Epidural anesthesia with local anesthetics appears to bypass this inhibition, thus reducing the duration of POI. The use of epidural opioids, however, does not reduce the duration of POI despite their analgesic effects.[27-30] In addition, inflammation secondary to surgery provides a causative factor in POI. Inflammatory mediators may have a direct effect on intestinal motility, with the severity of ileus directly correlating to the degree of intestinal inflammatory.[18]

Current Management of POI and OBD

Current treatment approaches for the management of OBD and POI have met with limited success in relieving patient symptoms. Given that laxatives, nutritional modifications (e.g., increased intake of fiber and fluids), and increased mobilization are the standard of care for treatment of functional or simple constipation, these interventions have also been applied for the management of OBD. However, as the underlying pathogenesis of OBD represents a complex constellation of symptoms consequent to the inhibitory effects of opioids on neural and secretory activity, protocols developed for the treatment of simple constipation have limited efficacy for the management of OBD.[7,31,32] Although the treatment of POI often incorporates use of nasogastric suction, early mobilization, early enteral feeding, and prokinetic agents, clinical trials evaluating the use of these treatments for POI have not demonstrated a consistent effect on gastrointestinal motility and patient comfort.[33-45] Epidural local anesthetics and the use of less invasive laparoscopic procedures have demonstrated some effectiveness in decreasing the duration of POI, but they have shown equivocal effects on postoperative morbidity.[46] Opioid-sparing techniques, which incorporate lower dose levels of opioid analgesics with adjunctive NSAID (nonsteroidal anti-inflammatory drug) therapy, have also been evaluated for the treatment of both POI and OBD.[47,48] However, not only does long-term NSAID use carry associated risks of gastrointestinal and renal toxicity, this treatment approach often represents a trade-off of compromising optimum analgesia solely for the benefit of reducing unwanted adverse GI events. Clearly, newer treatment approaches are needed to manage the morbidity and health care costs associated with OBD and POI.

Given the predominance of peripheral opioid receptors in the pathogenesis of OBD and POI, there has been increasing interest in the use of selective antagonists for opioid receptors in the GI tract to potentially treat these disorders. Oral naloxone and nalmefene glucuronide have limited systemic bioavailability with oral administration, but clinical application has been limited by the observation that even minimally absorbed parent compound or pharmacologically active metabolites may cross the blood-brain barrier and antagonize centrally mediated analgesia.[49,50] Opioid antagonists with poor lipid solubility, such as alvimopan and methylnaltrexone, cannot readily cross the blood-brain barrier and therefore have peripherally re-stricted mechanisms of actions.[51-55] The potential benefit of these agents is their ability to antagonize opioid-mediated changes in GI motility without altering centrally mediated opioid effects, such as analgesia. Early clinical studies with methylnaltrexone showed prom-ise in its ability to reverse opioid-induced delays in GI transit time in volunteers without reversing analgesia or inducing symptoms of withdrawal.[51,52] The results of Phase II and Phase III studies examin-ing the use of alvimopan to normalize bowel function in patients with OBD and to reduce the severity and duration of POI are discussed herein.

PRECLINICAL DEVELOPMENT

Physical and Chemical Properties

Alvimopan (formerly known as LY246736, Eli Lilly & Co., and ADL 8-2698, Adolor Corporation) is a novel, oral, peripherally act-ing *trans*-3,4-dimethyl-4-(3-hydroxyphenyl) piperidine opioid an-tagonist with a high affinity for the mu opioid receptor (see Figure 11.1).[53,55] The moderately large molecular weight, zwitterionic form, and polarity of alvimopan inhibit crossing of the blood-brain barrier and potential antagonism of opioid-induced central nervous system (CNS) effects.[53,54]

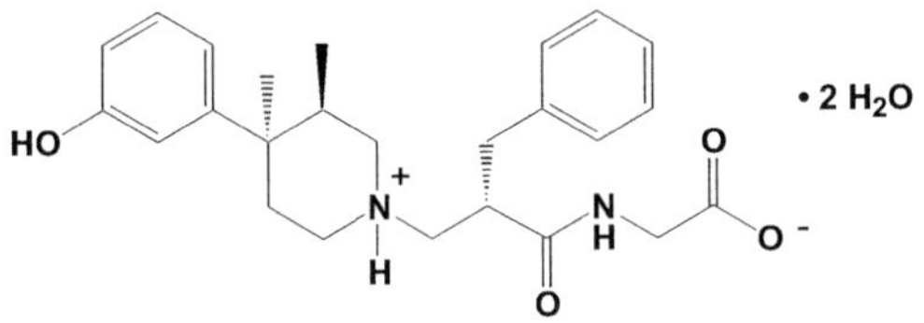

Alvimopan (Entereg, ADL 8-2698)

- [[2(S)-[[4(R)-)3-hydroxyphenyl)-3(R),4-dimethyl-1-piperidinyl]methyl]-1-oxo-3-phenylpropyl]amino]acetic acid dihydrate

- Small molecule ($C_{25}H_{32}N_2O_4 \cdot 2H_2O$); totally synthetic

- MW: 460.6

FIGURE 11.1. Structure of alvimopan (Entereg).

Preclinical Pharmacology

Alvimopan has been demonstrated to be a potent antagonist of mu opioid receptors both in vitro and in vivo. In radioligand-binding assays, alvimopan has a high affinity for the mu opioid receptor ($K_i =$ 0.77 nM) and lower affinities for delta ($K_i = 4.4$ nM) and kappa ($K_i =$ 40 nM) receptors.[53,54] Alvimopan is approximately fivefold more potent in inhibiting the mu opioid receptor than naloxone ($K_i = 3.7$ nM)[54] and approximately 68-fold more potent than methylnaltrexone ($K_i = 68$ nM).[56] Alvimopan does not demonstrate any biologically relevant affinity for nonopioid receptors such as the adrenergic, serotonergic, dopaminergic, histaminic, or muscarinic receptors.[54]

Administered orally or intravenously (IV) in animals, alvimopan shows strong preferential inhibition of the peripheral versus central mu opioid receptors. Peripheral antagonist activity was evaluated by induction of diarrhea in morphine-dependent mice, and central antagonist activity was measured by antagonism of morphine-induced analgesia in mice. Following IV administration, alvimopan is approximately 200 times more potent at blocking peripheral versus central mu receptors.[54] Alvimopan antagonizes centrally mediated morphine-induced analgesia only at relatively high doses, requiring very high plasma concentrations to cross the blood-brain barrier. In time-response studies, alvimopan also reversed morphine-induced constipation in the mouse charcoal meal test for at least eight hours without antagonizing morphine's actions in the central nervous system, as evaluated by the absence of withdrawal-mediated jumping behavior in morphine-dependent mice.[54] A summary of the preclinical pharmacology of alvimopan versus naloxone is shown in Table 11.1.[54]

Preclinical Pharmacokinetics and Metabolism

Preclinical models suggest that plasma concentrations of alvimopan are dose dependent with IV administration. In dogs and rabbits, the $t_{1/2}$ in serum is approximately ten minutes after IV administration, with no accumulation in the plasma compartment.[54] Over a 30-day period, peak plasma levels in dogs were proportional to IV doses and exceeded 4,000 ng/mL following a 2 mg/kg IV dose. However, in these preclinical models, alvimopan appeared to be poorly absorbed with oral administration. With oral doses up to 100 mg/kg, only low

TABLE 11.1. Gastrointestinal effects of opioid antagonists in preclinical pharmacology models.

Assay	Alvimopan	Naloxone
Opioid receptor binding (K_i)		
mu ([^{3}H]naloxone), nM	0.77	3.7
delta ([^{3}H]DADLE), nM	4.4	32
kappa ([^{3}H]EKC), n^m	40	66
Opioid receptor antagonist pA_2 values in guinea pig ileum (mu, kappa) or rat vas deferens (delta)		
mu (DAMGO)	9.7	8.5
delta (DPDPE)	8.7	7.3
kappa (U-69, 593)	7.8	7.7
Precipitation of diarrhea in morphine-dependent mice, mg/kg^a	0.04 (IV)	0.31 (SC)
Antagonism of morphine analgesia in mice, mg/kg^b	9.0 (IV)	1.5 (SC)

Source: Adapted with permission from Zimmerman DM, Gidda JS, Cantrell BE. LY246736 dihydrate μ opioid receptor antagonist. *Drugs of the Future* 1994; 19:1078-1083. Reprinted with permission.

K_i = inhibition constant; pA_2 = Log^{-1} measure of antagonist potency; DADLE = D-Ala^2-D-Leu^5-enkephalin; DAMGO = Tyr-D-Ala-Gly-MePhe-NH-(CH$_2$)$_2$OH; DPDPE = D-Pen^2-D-Pen^5-enkephalin; EKC = ethylketocyclazocine; IV = intravenous; SC = subcutaneous.

^{a}Dose that precipitated diarrhea in 50 percent of mice.
^{b}Dose that reduced the inhibition of writhing by 50 percent.

plasma concentrations (mean C_{max} = 92.9 ng/mL) were observed, resulting in an oral bioavailability of approximately 0.03 percent.[54]

The strong specificity of alvimopan for peripheral mu opioid receptors and low permeability across the blood-brain barrier has been demonstrated in whole-body autoradiography studies in rats (see Figure 11.2).[55] Following IV administration, alvimopan could be seen distributed to most parts of the rat body, with the exception of the spinal cord and brain. Similar findings were reported with oral administration in autoradiographic studies by Zimmerman et al.[54] In the latter study, the majority of radiolabel associated with an orally administered dose of [^{14}C]alvimopan in rats was found within the GI tract, much of it within the gut wall. Minimal absorption was reported with limited distribution to extraintestinal tissues.

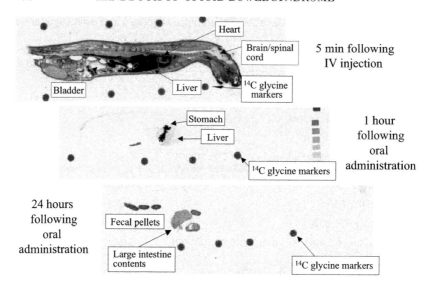

FIGURE 11.2. Whole body autoradiographs of rats administered [14C]alvimopan. Rats received oral or IV doses containing 20 μCi/kg [14C]alvimopan. (A) autoradiogram five minutes after 2.0 mg/kg IV shows distribution of [14C] throughout the body with the exception of the brain or spinal cord; (B) autoradiogram at one hour after a 200 mg/kg PO dose of alvimopan; and (C) autoradiogram at 24 hours after a 200 mg/kg PO dose of alvimopan. Overall, radiograms show that the [14C] label is restricted to the GI tract at 1 to 24 hours after oral dosing in rats. *Source:* Reprinted from *American Journal of Surgery,* 182(5A suppl), Schmidt WK, Alvimopan (ADL 8-2698) is a novel peripheral opioid antagonist, S27-S38, Copyright 2001, with permission from Excerpta Medica, Inc.

Preclinical Safety and Toxicity

In preclinical models, alvimopan was generally well tolerated; acute and subacute toxicology studies have shown that alvimopan has a large therapeutic index.[54] Oral doses up to 200 mg/kg in rats and 100 mg/kg in dogs were evaluated in six-month safety studies, with no notable toxicologic findings. In addition, no reproductive or developmental safety issues were identified from in vitro and in vivo studies in animals.[54,55]

CLINICAL DEVELOPMENT

Based on the preclinical in vitro and in vivo studies that demonstrated the high specificity of alvimopan for the mu opioid receptor and its peripheral restriction outside of the CNS, several Phase I studies were conducted in humans to characterize the safety and tolerability of orally administered alvimopan in normal human volunteers, as well as the effects of alvimopan on GI motility and transit time following the administration of systemic opioids. Additional studies established whether alvimopan would act centrally to limit the analgesia or pupillary constriction associated with opioid therapy.

Antagonism of Opioid-Induced Delay of Upper Gastrointestinal Transit

The effect of alvimopan on human GI transit was evaluated in an early clinical trial of eight healthy volunteers. This study evaluated whether alvimopan could reverse or prevent the inhibitory GI activity of loperamide, a mu opioid agonist indicated for the treatment of diarrhea, as measured by transit of radio-opaque markers in the colon.[55] In this double-blind, placebo-controlled, balanced crossover study, 8 men 28 to 54 years of age were administered either loperamide 8 mg b.i.d. or placebo. As expected, loperamide inhibited GI transit, causing a twofold increase in colonic transit time compared with the control group ($p < 0.01$) (see Figure 11.3). The subgroup of individuals who received loperamide were also administered additional doses of placebo or alvimopan 2.4 or 24 mg three times daily over the course of four days. Alvimopan completely prevented the loperamide-induced changes in GI transit at both 2.4 and 24 mg t.i.d.[55,57]

Alvimopan reversal of morphine-induced delays in upper GI transit (oral-cecal transit time) was evaluated as a measure of alvimopan's ability to protect against morphine's inhibitory effects on upper GI transit, as measured by the lactulose hydrogen breath test.[58,59] In a double-blind, placebo-controlled, balanced crossover study of 14 healthy volunteers, 7 men and 7 women were administered 1 of 3 treatments on 3 separate days: oral and IV placebo, oral placebo and IV morphine (0.05 mg/kg), and oral alvimopan (4 mg) and IV morphine (0.05 mg/kg). Intravenous morphine alone increased GI transit time from 69 to 103 minutes ($p = 0.005$) (see Figure 11.4). Coadmin-

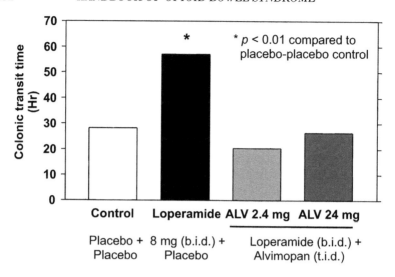

FIGURE 11.3. Alvimopan reverses delay of gastrointestinal transit induced by loperamide. Radio-opaque markers were administered orally on the morning of the first three treatment days of each cycle; the location of the markers was determined via abdominal X-ray on the fourth to fifth treatment day to determine colonic transit time. *Source:* Reprinted from *American Journal of Surgery,* 182(5A suppl), Schmidt WK, Alvimopan (ADL 8-2698) is a novel peripheral opioid antagonist, S27-S38, Copyright 2001, with permission from Excerpta Medica, Inc.

istration of oral alvimopan prevented the morphine-induced delay in GI transit time ($p = 0.004$), producing transit times similar to those of baseline.

Antagonism of Opioid-Induced Delay of Lower GI Transit and Lack of Analgesic Antagonism

In preclinical models, administration of alvimopan during opioid therapy normalizes bowel motility and GI transit time without reversing centrally mediated opioid effects. The ability of alvimopan to reverse morphine-induced delays in lower GI transit without antagonizing opioid effects in the CNS was evaluated in a Phase I, randomized, placebo-controlled, crossover trial involving 13 healthy volunteers.[55,60] GI transit was measured using radio-opaque markers. Individuals received either placebo or alvimopan 3 mg orally t.i.d. and morphine

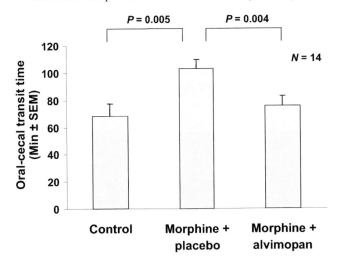

FIGURE 11.4. Alvimopan prevents morphine-induced delay in oral-cecal transit time. Oral-cecal transit time was measured by the lactulose hydrogen breath test procedure. *Source:* Reprinted from *American Journal of Surgery*, 182(5A suppl), Schmidt WK, Alvimopan (ADL 8-2698) is a novel peripheral opioid antagonist, S27-S38, Copyright 2001, with permission from Excerpta Medica, Inc.

30 mg orally b.i.d. for four days. This was followed by a washout period of one week, and then four days of the crossover treatment. Efficacy assessment occurred after each treatment period and included GI transit (as measured by the weighted sum of radio-opaque marker transit scores in the colon), and measures of CNS opioid antagonism (cold pressor pain scores and pupillary size). Coadministration of alvimopan with morphine was associated with a significantly faster GI transit time ($p < 0.05$), increased number of stools ($p < 0.05$), and increased stool weight ($p < 0.05$) as compared with placebo. In contrast, coadministration of alvimopan did not antagonize the central effects of morphine as shown by its failure to change the magnitude of pupil constriction with morphine administration.[55,60]

Liu et al.[59] assessed the effects of alvimopan reversal of morphine-induced analgesia and pupillary constriction in 45 patients who underwent dental surgery. Patients were randomly assigned in a double-blind fashion to one of three treatment groups ($n = 15$ per group): oral alvimopan (total = 4 mg) and IV morphine 0.15 mg/kg, oral placebo and IV morphine 0.15 mg/kg, or oral placebo and IV placebo. Morphine significantly reduced visual analog scale (VAS) pain scores and categorical pain scores, and increased pain relief scores. Administration of alvimopan before and after surgery did not affect either pain scores (see Figure 11.5) or morphine-induced pupillary constriction.[59]

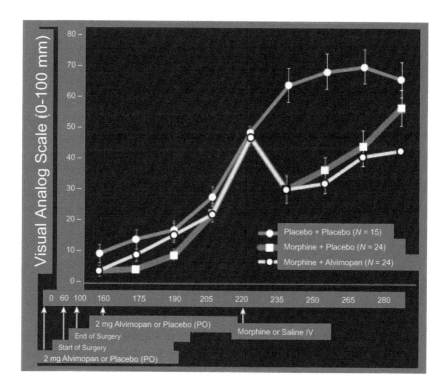

FIGURE 11.5. Alvimopan does not reverse morphine analgesia in healthy volunteers undergoing third molar extraction. Patients received two 2 mg oral doses of alvimopan (administered 60 minutes before surgery and again 60 minutes after surgery; 4 mg total dose) or placebo along with IV morphine (0.15 mg/kg) or saline in a double-blind procedure. Morphine or saline doses were administered after patients reported moderate or severe pain (mean visual analog scale score = 50). Morphine with and without alvimopan decreased pain scores and was significantly different from the placebo-saline group ($p < 0.002$). *Source:* Reprinted from *American Journal of Surgery,* 182(5A suppl), Schmidt WK, Alvimopan (ADL 8-2698) is a novel peripheral opioid antagonist, S27-S38, Copyright 2001, with permission from Excerpta Medica, Inc.

Clinical Safety and Tolerability

A Phase I, dose-escalating study evaluated the clinical safety and dose-related side effects of alvimopan in 44 healthy volunteers.[55] In a single-center, double-blind, placebo-controlled trial, healthy human volunteers were randomized to receive placebo ($n = 5$) or alvimopan 0.25, 0.5, 2.0, 6.0, or 18.0 mg t.i.d. ($n = 4, 11, 9, 9$, and 6, respectively; total doses = 0.75 to 54 mg/day), beginning with a three-week screening period followed by oral dosing for four consecutive days. The most common adverse events reported by subjects administered alvimopan were dose related, occurring at total daily doses of 18 mg and higher, and included abdominal pain (31 percent), flatulence (31 percent), and diarrhea (21 percent). Nausea, polyuria, and nervousness also were reported to a lesser degree. These adverse events occurred infrequently at lower doses. One subject randomized to receive 18 mg t.i.d. withdrew during the second day of dosing due to abdominal pain, nausea, and diarrhea after receiving a total dose of 72 mg. No serious adverse events were reported. Abnormal laboratory values were reported by two patients; both patients had clinically significant elevations in liver function tests (AST, ALT, and LDH; maximum increases of 2.5 to 4.0 ULN) that subsequently returned to baseline without intervention. No dose-related hepatotoxicity was reported. Overall, this study demonstrated that alvimopan is generally well tolerated at doses up to 54 mg/day for four days with no occurrence of serious adverse events or hepatotoxicity.

No serious adverse events were reported in Phase I and Phase II studies of patients treated with alvimopan for OBD or POI, with the exception of localized GI side effects (abdominal cramps, diarrhea, nausea, vomiting) experienced by some chronic opioid patients receiving apparently supramaximal doses (3 mg or higher) of alvimopan for the OBD indication.

Clinical Trials in POI

The ability of alvimopan to accelerate postoperative recovery of GI function and decrease hospital stay was initially evaluated in a single-center Phase II trial.[61] In this randomized, placebo-controlled trial, 78 patients undergoing laparotomy for hysterectomy ($n = 63$) or partial colectomy ($n = 15$) were assigned to receive alvimopan 1 mg

($n = 26$), alvimopan 6 mg ($n = 26$), or placebo ($n = 26$) orally two hours before surgery, and then b.i.d. postoperatively until the first occurrence of bowel movement, hospital discharge, or for a maximum of seven days, whichever occurred first. The mean age of the patients was approximately 53 years, and most (89 percent) were women. Although all patients received general anesthesia, the specific anesthetic and surgical management protocol were not specified by study protocol. The duration of surgery did not differ among treatment groups. For postoperative pain management, all patients received either morphine sulfate or meperidine hydrochloride via IV patient-controlled analgesia.

The primary efficacy outcomes were prospectively defined as time to first flatus, time to first bowel movement, and time to readiness for hospital discharge. Secondary end points were the time to first toleration of liquids, time to first toleration of solid foods, time to actual discharge, and VAS scores for nausea, abdominal cramping, itching, and pain. Median time to each end point was assessed by Kaplan-Meier log-rank analysis.

For patients who received 6 mg alvimopan b.i.d., median time to first passage of flatus was accelerated by 0.9 days compared with placebo ($p = 0.03$), median time to first bowel movement was accelerated by 1.7 days compared with placebo ($p = 0.01$), and median time to readiness for discharge was accelerated by approximately one day (23 hours) compared with placebo ($p = 0.03$).[61] The results for 1 mg alvimopan were intermediate but not statistically different from placebo.

Alvimopan 6 mg also showed statistical superiority over placebo for secondary outcomes. Compared with placebo, alvimopan 6 mg significantly accelerated median time to toleration of first solid food by 1.4 days ($p < 0.001$), and median time to actual discharge by 1.2 days ($p < 0.001$) compared with placebo. Similar results were obtained for mean response times (see Figure 11.6). Patients treated with 6 mg alvimopan also reported significantly less postoperative nausea and vomiting compared with placebo (see Figure 11.7) and did not show antagonism of opioid analgesia (see Figure 11.8).

Moreover, alvimopan did not appear to cross the blood-brain barrier and antagonize postoperative pain management (see Table 11.2). Morphine dose equivalents administered by patient-controlled analgesia were equivalent among the three study groups ($p = 0.91$), im-

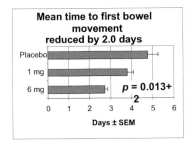

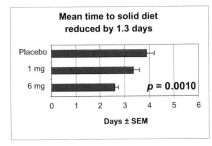

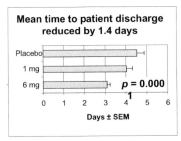

- **Bowel function normalized more rapidly**
- **Solid food tolerated earlier**
- **Patients discharged sooner**

FIGURE 11.6. Alvimopan accelerates recovery of bowel function and shortens hospital stay after laparotomy. Patients ($n = 78$) who underwent laparotomy were administered 1 mg alvimopan, 6 mg alvimopan, or placebo two hours before surgery, then b.i.d. starting on postoperative day 1 until hospital discharge. Overall log-rank test p values (*) and individual p values (†) are given for 6 mg alvimopan versus placebo. (A) Mean time to first bowel movement was accelerated by 2.0 days (*$p = 0.0132$; †$p = 0.01$); (B) mean time to toleration of solid food was accelerated by 1.3 days (*$p = 0.0001$; †$p = 0.001$); and (C) mean time to hospital discharge was accelerated by 1.4 days (*$p = 0.0001$; †$p = 0.001$). *Source:* Reprinted from *American Journal of Surgery,* 182(5A suppl), Schmidt WK, Alvimopan (ADL 8-2698) is a novel peripheral opioid antagonist, S27-S38, Copyright 2001, with permission from Excerpta Medica, Inc.

plying no antagonism of analgesia. Maximal VAS scores for pain and itching were also similar across treatment groups.

Overall, in this Phase II, placebo-controlled study, 6 mg alvimopan b.i.d. significantly accelerated time to recovery of GI function and significantly decreased the duration of hospitalization, without antagonizing postoperative pain management in patients undergoing abdominal surgery.[61]

The Phase III POI clinical development program included one safety and three efficacy clinical studies with a total of 2,146 patients.[56] Summary results from all 3 recently completed efficacy

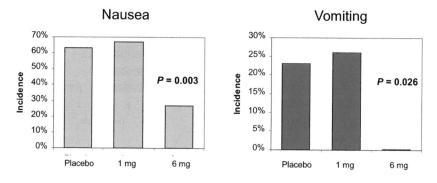

FIGURE 11.7. Alvimopan significantly reduced nausea and vomiting in 78 patients undergoing either hysterectomy or partial colectomy. Individual *P* values for 6 mg alvimopan versus placebo are shown. *Source:* Reprinted from *American Journal of Surgery,* 182(5A suppl), Schmidt WK, Alvimopan (ADL 8-2698) is a novel peripheral opioid antagonist, S27-S38, Copyright 2001, with permission from Excerpta Medica, Inc.

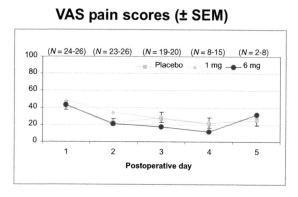

FIGURE 11.8. Alvimopan does not antagonize analgesia in postoperative ileus. Number of patients in each dose group are shown for each postoperative day. Morphine consumption represents patient-controlled analgesia doses of morphine or morphine-equivalent doses of meperidine. *Source:* Reprinted from *American Journal of Surgery,* 182(5A suppl), Schmidt WK, Alvimopan (ADL 8-2698) is a novel peripheral opioid antagonist, S27-S38, Copyright 2001, with permission from Excerpta Medica, Inc.

TABLE 11.2. Alvimopan did not antagonize postoperative analgesia in 78 patients undergoing hysterectomy or partial colectomy.

		1 mg Alvimopan (*n* = 26)	6 mg Alvimopan (*n* = 26)	
Cumulative morphine sulfate, mg	71 ± 58	70 ± 61	71 ± 52	0.91
Maximal VAS pain score	54 ± 25	62 ± 24	53 ± 21	0.30
Maximal VAS itching score	16 ± 28	25 ± 29	28 ± 36	0.48

Source: Adapted with permission from Taguchi A, Sharma N, Saleem RM, et al. Selective postoperative inhibition of gastrointestinal opioid receptors. *N Engl J Med* 2001;345:935-40.
Note: VAS = visual analog scale; values are mean ± standard deviation.

studies showed that 6 and 12 mg doses of alvimopan accelerated time to GI recovery (composite primary end point, defined as passage of either first flatus or stool and toleration of a solid diet). The 6 mg dose was statistically different from placebo ($p < 0.01$, $p < 0.05$) in two trials with a trend toward significance in the third trial. The 12 mg dose was statistically significant from placebo in one trial ($p < 0.01$), with a trend toward significance in two other trials. Mean time to hospital discharge order written was significantly improved by approximately 8 to 20 hours across the three studies. Fewer patients were rehospitalized within 10 days postdischarge across all alvimopan treatment groups (range = 2.7 to 5.3 percent) compared to the 3 placebo groups (range = 6.7 to 8.5 percent) and fewer patients required reinsertion of nasogastric tubes following surgery (alvimopan treatment groups = 2.1 to 8.4 percent; placebo groups = 6.9 to 14.8 percent). Alvimopan was generally well tolerated; nausea, vomiting, hypotension, and pruritus were the most frequently observed adverse events across the three efficacy studies and occurred with apparently similar frequencies among the placebo and alvimopan treatment groups.[56] Further studies are planned or under way to evaluate the safety and efficacy of alvimopan in additional populations receiving short postoperative courses of opioid analgesics.

Clinical Trials in OBD

Because preliminary findings showed that alvimopan could prevent or reverse the GI effects of opioids without affecting analgesia in normal subjects, alvimopan was evaluated in Phase II trials of 101 patients with symptoms of OBD who were on long-term opioid therapy for chronic pain ($n = 67$) or methadone for opioid addiction ($n = 34$).[55] Opioid therapy for treatment of chronic pain was variable and consisted of different doses of hydrocodone and acetaminophen (APAP), oxycodone and APAP, codeine and APAP, fentanyl, extended-release oral morphine, extended-release oxycodone, tramadol, meperidine, or propoxyphene. Opioid-addicted patients received methadone 40 to 100 mg/day. The duration of opioid therapy in these patients ranged from one week to ten or more years. Patients were enrolled into one of two treatment arms.

The first study was a parallel-group, single-dose study design in which 75 patients received either placebo or alvimopan 0.5, 1.5, or 3.0 mg orally. Efficacy analysis involved both the incidence of bowel movements within 12 hours of the single dose and the weight of stool. Approximately 20 to 22 patients received each dose of alvimopan 0, 0.5, or 1.5 mg; only 11 patients received the 3.0 mg dose before it was discontinued due to an increased incidence of diarrhea, nausea, severe abdominal cramping, and vomiting in some patients. Alvimopan significantly increased the incidence of bowel movements and stool weight within 12 hours of dosing in a dose-dependent manner (see Figure 11.9). These increases were significantly different from placebo for all doses of alvimopan tested. Patients taking alvimopan reported dose-related decreases in the incidence of hard, dry stool as well as decreases in the incidence of moderate to severe straining. The maximum response after a single dose of alvimopan was seen within approximately 4 hours following the highest dose (3 mg) of alvimopan and 7 hours following the lowest dose (0.5 mg) (see Figure 11.10). Patient satisfaction with bowel function was rated significantly higher for patients treated with all doses of alvimopan compared with placebo (see Figure 11.11). Alvimopan was well tolerated. Adverse events were minimal, particularly at the 0.5 and 1.5 mg doses of alvimopan. A small number of patients receiving alvimopan 3 mg (the highest dose) reported loose stools, cramps, and/or diarrhea, possibly indicating a localized gut-specific opioid withdrawal. No

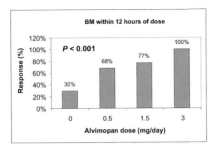
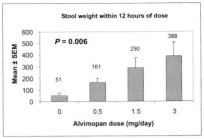

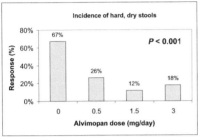
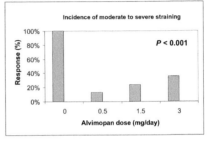

FIGURE 11.9. Alvimopan significantly increased the incidence of bowel movements within 12 hours of a single dose in patients with opioid bowel dysfunction (*n* = 75) who were receiving stable doses of opioid therapy for nonmalignant chronic pain or methadone maintenance. (A) Percentage of patients with a bowel movement within 12 hours of dosing (*p* < 0.001 overall treatment differences); (B) stool weight within 12 hours of dosing (*p* < 0.001 overall treatment differences); (C) incidence of hard, dry stools (*p* < 0.001 overall treatment differences); and (D) incidence of moderate to severe straining upon defecation (*p* < 0.001 overall treatment differences). Overall treatment *p* values are shown. *Source:* Reprinted from *American Journal of Surgery,* 182(5A suppl), Schmidt WK, Alvimopan (ADL 8-2698) is a novel peripheral opioid antagonist, S27-S38, Copyright 2001, with permission from Excerpta Medica, Inc.

patients exhibited symptoms of CNS opioid withdrawal or reversal of analgesia. Similar gut-specific withdrawal effects were observed in one opioid-dependent chronic pain patient receiving the 3 mg dose in a small (*n* = 7) open-label dose-ranging pilot study.[62]

The second study involved a progressive dosing "forced titration" study of 26 patients on stable, long-term opioid therapy for chronic nonmalignant pain, in which patients were administered either placebo (*n* = 9) or increasing once-daily doses of alvimopan (*n* = 17) across 4 days (alvimopan 0.5, 1.5, 3.0, or 4.5 mg on days 1 to 4,

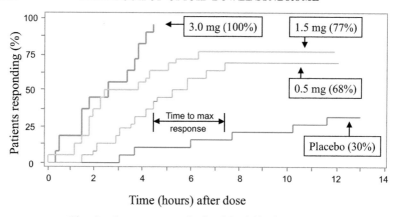

Single-dose protocol, double-blind, $N = 75$

FIGURE 11.10. Alvimopan significantly and dose dependently increases time to first bowel movement in chronic opioid patients. Patients were administered single doses of placebo ($n = 20$), alvimopan 0.5 mg ($n = 22$), alvimopan 1.5 mg ($n = 22$), or alvimopan 3.0 mg ($n = 11$). *Source:* Reprinted from *American Journal of Surgery*, 182(5A suppl), Schmidt WK, Alvimopan (ADL 8-2698) is a novel peripheral opioid antagonist, S27-S38, Copyright 2001, with permission from Excerpta Medica, Inc.

respectively).[55,63] In patients treated with alvimopan, mean stool weight per day increased on successive study days up until day 3, whereas mean daily stool weight for patients treated with placebo remained constant and significantly lower (see Figure 11.12). The slight reduction in mean stool weight on day 4 from that observed on day 3 in patients treated with alvimopan was attributed to increased elimination of retained constipation-related stool on the previous 3 days and subsequent return to more normal stool volume by the fourth day. Again, patients exhibited no symptoms of opioid withdrawal or antagonism of opioid-mediated analgesia.

Summary results of a Phase III trial of alvimopan in patients with opioid bowel dysfunction were announced in April 2002.[56] A total of 168 nonmalignant pain or opioid pharmacotherapy patients who had been on chronic opioid therapy for at least 1 month and who suffered from opioid bowel dysfunction received once-daily oral dosing of either 0.5 mg or 1 mg alvimopan or placebo for 21 consecutive days.

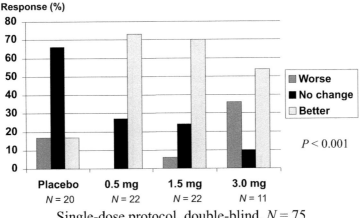

Single-dose protocol, double-blind, $N = 75$

FIGURE 11.11. Alvimopan significantly increases patient overall satisfaction with bowel movements in patients on chronic opioid therapy. $N = 20$ to 22 subjects per dose except in the 3.0 mg group ($n = 11$). Further details are presented with Figure 11.9; $p < 0.001$ for overall treatment with alvimopan. *Source:* Reprinted from *American Journal of Surgery,* 182(5A suppl), Schmidt WK, Alvimopan (ADL 8-2698) is a novel peripheral opioid antagonist, S27-S38, Copyright 2001, with permission from Excerpta Medica, Inc.

For the primary end point, both doses of alvimopan significantly increased the percentage of patients who had a bowel movement within eight hours of each daily dose. On average, patients treated with alvimopan were significantly more likely to have a bowel movement within eight hours of dosing compared with placebo. Across the 21-day study period, only 29 percent of patients treated with placebo experienced a bowel movement within 8 hours of dosing, compared with 43 percent of patients treated with alvimopan 0.5 mg ($p < 0.001$ versus placebo) and 54 percent of patients treated with alvimopan 1 mg ($p < 0.001$ versus placebo). Alvimopan was well tolerated in this patient population; the most commonly reported adverse events were transient and dose related, and included diarrhea, abdominal cramps, nausea, and vomiting.

Overall, alvimopan has been shown to improve bowel function in patients treated with long-term opioid therapy for chronic pain and in patients undergoing methadone therapy for the pharmacotherapy

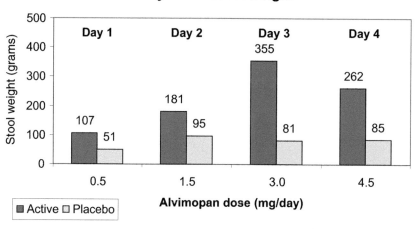

FIGURE 11.12. Alvimopan significantly increases mean daily stool weight with progressive doses administered across 4 days in 26 patients receiving long-term stable opioid therapy for chronic nonmalignant pain; $p = 0.002$ for overall effect of alvimopan treatment versus placebo. *Source:* Reprinted from *American Journal of Surgery,* 182(5A suppl), Schmidt WK, Alvimopan (ADL 8-2698) is a novel peripheral opioid antagonist, S27-S38, Copyright 2001, with permission from Excerpta Medica, Inc.

of opioid addiction. Alvimopan is a peripherally acting mu opioid antagonist with actions selective for the GI tract, as demonstrated by a lack of inhibition of centrally mediated opioid effects. Further studies are planned to evaluate the safety and durability of alvimopan efficacy in OBD patients with longer-term treatments and in patients with malignancy-associated pain.

SUMMARY

Regulation of GI motility involves complex interactions between neural input, smooth muscle contraction, water and electrolyte flux across the mucous membrane, and the effects of neurohormonal and inflammatory mediators. It is clear that the coordination of this system is significantly disrupted in patients with OBD and POI. Stimulation of opioid receptors in the enteric and central nervous system create an inhibitory effect on the propulsive and secretory aspects of GI function that does not decrease with chronic administration of opioids. Moreover, the effects of opioids on the GI tract may be sufficiently severe to become dose limiting and therefore interfere with the attainment of optimal analgesia. Treatment approaches that can minimize these adverse effects without compromising analgesia remain a critical unmet medical need.

Alvimopan is a novel peripherally acting opioid antagonist that blocks the effects of opioids on the GI tract without compromising pain relief. Alvimopan has low and variable systemic absorption, with activity selective to the GI tract after oral administration. The affinity of alvimopan for the mu opioid receptor is high, approximately 68 times that of methylnaltrexone and fivefold higher than naloxone.

In clinical trials, alvimopan accelerated the return of GI function after surgery in opioid-naive patients, and reversed opioid-induced constipation and other symptoms of OBD such as nausea, vomiting, and abdominal cramping and bloating in opioid-tolerant patients. Alvimopan appears to be well tolerated with adverse effects similar to those of placebo. Adverse events that occur more frequently in patients treated with alvimopan compared with placebo are generally transient and dose related; symptoms include mild to moderate nausea, vomiting, and diarrhea. In conclusion, the results of multiple clinical studies suggest that alvimopan may treat many of the symptoms of OBD and accelerate recovery of GI function following major abdominal surgery without affecting opioid analgesia for the management of POI and OBD.

Editor's Note

Since completion of this chapter, Adolor Corporation (www.adolor.com) and GSK (GlaxoSmithKline, www.gsk.com) have completed the following clinical studies on alvimopan (or Entereg).

The alvimopan postoperative ileus Phase 3 clinical program, including four clinical trials, enrolled over 2,100 subjects in total. The primary endpoint in the studies was time to recovery of gastrointestinal function, as defined by time to tolerability of solid foods and time to first flatus or first bowel movement, whichever occurred last. Data from one of these trials in over 500 patients were published in *Ann. Surg.* (240:728-34; 2004) showing that alvimopan significantly accelerated gastrointestinal recovery in patients undergoing laparotomy for bowel resection or radical hysterectomy; hospital discharge orders were written for patients taking 12 mg of alvimopan approximately one day earlier as compared with those taking placebo. Adolor completed submission of a New Drug Application to the Food and Drug Administration for use of Entereg capsules in postoperative ileus on June 28, 2004.

GSK has completed a Phase 2b study of alvimopan for the treatment of opioid-induced bowel dysfunction (OBD), which results from the use of opioids in patients suffering from chronic pain. This study, in 522 non-cancer patients with OBD, showed that oral alvimopan 0.5 to 1.0 mg achieved statistically significant effects on increasing the frequency of spontaneous bowel movements and also improvements in straining, stool consistency, and incomplete evacuation compared with placebo. The incidence of patients reporting adverse events was numerically similar between treatment and placebo groups. There was no evidence of antagonism of opioid analgesia based upon pain intensity scores and opioid consumption.

NOTES

1. Gutstein HB, Akil H. Opioid analgesics. In Hardman JG, Limbird LE, Gilman AG (eds.), *Goodman & Gilman's the pharmacological basis of therapeutics*. 10th ed. New York: McGraw-Hill Medical Publishing Division; 2001:569-619.

2. Bagnol D, Mansour A, Akil H, Watson SJ. Cellular localization and distribution of the cloned mu and kappa opioid receptors in rat gastrointestinal tract. *Neuroscience* 1997;81:579-591.

3. Fickel J, Bagnol D, Watson SJ, Akil H. Opioid receptor expression in the rat gastrointestinal tract: A quantitative study with comparison to the brain. *Brain Res Mol Brain Res* 1997;46:1-8.

4. De Luca A, Coupar IM. Insights into opioid action in the intestinal tract. *Pharmacol Ther* 1996;69:103-115.

5. Shook JE, Pelton JT, Hruby VJ, Burks TF. Peptide opioid antagonist separates peripheral and central opioid antitransit effects. *J Pharmacol Exp Ther* 1987;243:492-500.

6. Friedman JD, Dello Buono FA. Opioid antagonists in the treatment of opioid-induced constipation and pruritus. *Ann Pharmacother* 2001;35:85-91.

7. Pappagallo M. Incidence, prevalence, and management of opioid bowel dysfunction. *Am J Surg* 2001;182(5A Suppl):11S-18S.

8. Azodo IA, Ehrenpreis ED. Alvimopan (Adolor/GlaxoSmithKline). *Curr Opin Investig Drugs* 2002;3:1496-1501.

9. Kaufman PN, Krevsky B, Malmud LS, Maurer AH, Somers MB, Siegel JA, Fisher RS. Role of opiate receptors in the regulation of colonic transit. *Gastroenterology* 1988;94:1351-1356.

10. Manara L, Bianchetti A. The central and peripheral influences of opioids on gastrointestinal propulsion. *Annu Rev Pharmacol Toxicol* 1985;25:249-2273.

11. Manara L, Bianchi G, Ferretti P, Tavani A. Inhibition of gastrointestinal transit by morphine in rats results primarily from direct drug action on gut opioid sites. *J Pharmacol Exp Ther* 1986;237:945-949.

12. Clevers GJ, Smout AJ. The natural course of postoperative ileus following abdominal surgery. *Neth J Surg* 1989;41:97-99.

13. Kehlet H. Postoperative ileus. *Gut* 2000;47(4 Suppl):iv85-86; discussion iv87.

14. Ogilvy AJ, Smith G. The gastrointestinal tract after anesthesia. *Eur J Anaesthesiol Suppl* 1995;10:35-42.

15. Schang JC, Hemond M, Hebert M, Pilote M. How does morphine work on colonic motility? An electromyographic study in the human left and sigmoid colon. *Life Sci* 1986;38:671-676.

16. Ferraz AA, Cowles VE, Condon RE, Carilli S, Ezberci F, Frantzides CT, Schulte WJ. Nonopioid analgesics shorten the duration of postoperative ileus. *Am Surg* 1995;61:1079-1083.

17. Holte K, Kehlet H. Postoperative ileus: A preventable event. *Br J Surg* 2000;87:1480-1493.

18. Kalff JC, Schraut WH, Simmons RL, Bauer AJ. Surgical manipulation of the gut elicits an intestinal muscularis inflammatory response resulting in postsurgical ileus. *Ann Surg* 1998;228:652-663.

19. Kehlet H. Acute pain control and accelerated postoperative surgical recovery. *Surg Clin North Am* 1999;79:431-443.

20. Prasad M, Matthews JB. Deflating postoperative ileus. *Gastroenterology* 1999;117:489-492.

21. Livingston EH, Passaro EP Jr. Postoperative ileus. *Dig Dis Sci* 1990;35:121-132.

22. Brix-Christensen V, Tonnesen E, Sanchez RG, Bilfinger TV, Stefano GB. Endogenous morphine levels increase following cardiac surgery as part of the anti-inflammatory response? *Int J Cardiol* 1997;62:191-197.

23. Brix-Christensen V, Goumon Y, Tonnesen E, Chew M, Bilfinger T, Stefano GB. Endogenous morphine is produced in response to cardiopulmonary bypass in neonatal pigs. *Acta Anaesthesiol Scand* 2000;44:1204-1208.

24. Kehlet H. Endogenous morphine—Another component and biological modifier of the response to surgical injury? *Acta Anaesthesiol Scand* 2000;44:1167-1168.

25. Yoshida S, Ohta J, Yamasaki K, Kamei H, Harada Y, Yahara T, Kaibara A, Ozaki K, Tajiri T, Shirouzu K. Effect of surgical stress on endogenous morphine and cytokine levels in the plasma after laparoscopic or open cholecystectomy. *Surg Endosc* 2000;14:137-140.

26. Frantzides CT, Cowles V, Salaymeh B, Tekin E, Condon RE. Morphine effects on human colonic myoelectric activity in the postoperative period. *Am J Surg* 1992;163:144-148.

27. Asantila R, Eklund P, Rosenberg PH. Continuous epidural infusion of bupivacaine and morphine for postoperative analgesia after hysterectomy. *Acta Anaesthesiol Scand* 1991;35:513-517.

28. Liu SS, Carpenter RL, Mackey DC, et al. Effects of perioperative analgesic technique on rate of recovery after colon surgery. *Anesthesiology* 1995;83:757-765.

29. Scheinin B, Asantila R, Orko R. The effect of bupivacaine and morphine on pain and bowel function after colonic surgery. *Acta Anaesthesiol Scand* 1987; 31:161-164.

30. Thoren T, Sundberg A, Wattwil M, Garvill JE, Jurgensen U. Effects of epidural bupivacaine and epidural morphine on bowel function and pain after hysterectomy. *Acta Anaesthesiol Scand* 1989;33:181-185.

31. Derby S, Portenoy RK. Assessment and management of opioid-induced constipation. In Portenoy RK, Bruera E (eds.), *Topics in palliative care* (Volume 1). New York: Oxford University Press; 1997:95-112.

32. Pappagallo M, Stewart W, Woods M. Constipation symptoms in long-term users of opioid analgesic therapy [abstract]. American Pain Society 18th Annual Meeting, October 21-24, 1999. Fort Lauderdale, FL. Abstract 750.

33. Fanning J, Yu-Brekke S. Prospective trial of aggressive postoperative bowel stimulation following radical hysterectomy. *Gynecol Oncol* 1999;73:412-414.

34. Waldhausen JH, Schirmer BD. The effect of ambulation on recovery from postoperative ileus. *Ann Surg* 1990;212:671-677.

35. Woods M. Postoperative ileus: Dogma versus data from bench to bedside. *Perspect Colon Rectal Surg* 2000;12:57-76.

36. Sangkhathat S, Patrapinyokul S, Tadyathikom K. Early enteral feeding after closure of colostomy in pediatric patients. *J Pediatr Surg* 2003;38:1516-1519.

37. Patolia DS, Hilliard RL, Toy EC, Baker B. Early feeding after cesarean: Randomized trial. *Obstet Gynecol* 2001;98:113-116.

38. Miedema BW, Schillie S, Simmons JW, Burgess SV, Liem T, Silver D. Small bowel motility and transit after aortic surgery. *J Vasc Surg* 2002;36:19-24.

39. Steed HL, Capstick V, Flood C, Schepansky A, Schulz J, Mayes DC. A randomized controlled trial of early versus "traditional" postoperative oral intake after major abdominal gynecologic surgery. *Am J Obstet Gynecol* 2002;186:861-865.

40. Hartsell PA, Frazee RC, Harrison JB, Smith RW. Early postoperative feeding after elective colorectal surgery. *Arch Surg* 1997;132:518-520.

41. Cheape JD, Wexner SD, James K, Jagelman DG. Does metoclopramide reduce the length of ileus after colorectal surgery? A prospective randomized trial. *Dis Colon Rectum* 1991;34:437-441.

42. Seta ML, Kale-Pradhan PB. Efficacy of metoclopramide in postoperative ileus after exploratory laparotomy. *Pharmacotherapy* 2001;21:1181-1186.

43. Roberts JP, Benson MJ, Rogers J, Deeks JJ, Wingate DL, Williams NS. Effect of cisapride on distal colonic motility in the early postoperative period following left colonic anastomosis. *Dis Colon Rectum* 1995;38:139-145.

44. Tollesson PO, Cassuto J, Rimback G, Faxen A, Bergman L, Mattsson E. Treatment of postoperative paralytic ileus with cisapride. *Scand J Gastroenterol* 1991;26:477-482.

45. Benson MJ, Roberts JP, Wingate DL, et al. Small bowel motility following major intra-abdominal surgery: The effects of opiates and rectal cisapride. *Gastroenterology* 1994;106:924-936.

46. Kehlet H, Holte K. Review of postoperative ileus. *Am J Surg* 2001;182(5A Suppl):3S-10S.

47. Tang J, Li S, White PF, Chen X, Wender RH, Quon R, Sloninsky A, Naruse R, Kariger R, Webb T, Norel E. Effect of parecoxib, a novel intravenous cyclo-

oxygenase type-2 inhibitor, on the postoperative opioid requirement and quality of pain control. *Anesthesiology* 2002;96:1305-1309.

48. Joishy SK, Walsh D. The opioid-sparing effects of intravenous ketorolac as an adjuvant analgesic in cancer pain: application in bone metastases and the opioid bowel syndrome. *J Pain Symptom Manage* 1998;16:334-339.

49. Cheskin LJ, Chami TN, Johnson RE, Jaffe JH. Assessment of nalmefene glucuronide as a selective gut opioid antagonist. *Drug Alcohol Depend* 1995; 39:151-154.

50. Meissner W, Schmidt U, Hartmann M, Kath R, Reinhart K. Oral naloxone reverses opioid-associated constipation. *Pain* 2000;84:105-109.

51. Yuan CS, Foss JF, O'Connor M, Osinski J, Roizen MF, Moss J. Effects of intravenous methylnaltrexone on opioid-induced gut motility and transit time changes in subjects receiving chronic methadone therapy: A pilot study. *Pain* 1999;83:631-635.

52. Yuan CS, Foss JF, O'Connor M, Osinki J, Karrison JM, Roizen MF. Methylnaltrexone for reversal of constipation due to chronic methadone use: A randomized controlled trial. *JAMA* 2000;283:367-372.

53. Zimmerman DM, Gidda JS, Cantrell BE, Schoepp DD, Johnson BG, Leander JD. Discovery of a potent, peripherally selective trans-3,4-dimethyl-4-(3-hydroxyphenyl)piperidine opioid antagonist for the treatment of gastrointestinal motility disorders. *J Med Chem* 1994;37:2262-2265.

54. Zimmerman DM, Gidda JS, Cantrell BE. LY246736 dihydrate μ opioid receptor antagonist. *Drugs of the Future* 1994;19:1078-1083.

55. Schmidt WK. Alvimopan (ADL 8-2698) is a novel peripheral opioid antagonist. *Am J Surg* 2001;182(5A Suppl):27S-38S.

56. Data on file. Adolor Corporation. Exton, PA. Topline phase III clinical study results available at <www.adolor.com>.

57. Callaghan JT, Cerimele B, Nowak TV, DeLong A, Nyhart E, Oldham S. Effect of the opioid antagonist LY246736 on gastrointestinal transit in human subjects. *Gastroenterology* 1998;114:G3015.

58. Hodgson PS, Liu SS, Carpenter RL. ADL 8-2698 prevents morphine inhibition of GI transit [abstract]. *Clin Pharmacol Ther* 2000;67:93.

59. Liu SS, Hodgson PS, Carpenter RL, Fricke JR Jr. ADL 8-2698, a *trans*-3,4-dimethyl-4-(3-hydroxyphenyl) piperidine, prevents gastrointestinal effects of intravenous morphine without affecting analgesia. *Clin Pharmacol Ther* 2001;69:66-71.

60. Barr WH, Nguyen P, Slattery M, Russell R, Carpenter RL. ADL 8-2698 reverses opioid induced delay in colonic transit [abstract]. *Clin Pharmacol Ther* 2000;67:91.

61. Taguchi A, Sharma N, Saleem RM, Sessler D, Carpenter RI, Seyedsadr M, Kurz A. Selective postoperative inhibition of gastrointestinal opioid receptors. *N Engl J Med* 2001;345:935-940.

62. Rauck RL, Southern JP, Carpenter RL. Use of alvimopan, a peripherally restricted μ-opioid antagonist, to speed gastrointestinal transit in patients with opioid induced bowel dysfunction [abstract]. Seattle, WA: IASP Press; 2002;550-551.

63. Paulson DM, Kennedy DT, Panebianco DI, Talluri K, Carpenter RL. A forced titration, dose ranging study of alvimopan for the reversal of opioid-induced bowel dysfunction [abstract]. Seattle, WA: IASP Press: 2002;197.

Index

Page numbers followed by the letter "f" indicate figures; those followed by the letter "t" indicate tables.

Order a copy of this book with this form or online at:
http://www.haworthpress.com/store/product.asp?sku=5523

HANDBOOK OF OPIOID BOWEL SYNDROME

_____ in hardbound at $79.95 (ISBN-13: 978-0-7890-2128-1; ISBN-10: 0-7890-2128-5)

_____ in softbound at $39.95 (ISBN-13: 978-0-7890-2129-8; ISBN-10: 0-7890-2129-3)

Or order online and use special offer code HEC25 in the shopping cart.

COST OF BOOKS_____

POSTAGE & HANDLING_____
(US: $4.00 for first book & $1.50
for each additional book)
(Outside US: $5.00 for first book
& $2.00 for each additional book)

SUBTOTAL_____

IN CANADA: ADD 7% GST_____

STATE TAX_____
(NJ, NY, OH, MN, CA, IL, IN, PA, & SD
residents, add appropriate local sales tax)

FINAL TOTAL_____
(If paying in Canadian funds,
convert using the current
exchange rate, UNESCO
coupons welcome)

☐ **BILL ME LATER:** (Bill-me option is good on
US/Canada/Mexico orders only; not good to
jobbers, wholesalers, or subscription agencies.)
☐ Check here if billing address is different from
shipping address and attach purchase order and
billing address information.

Signature_____

☐ **PAYMENT ENCLOSED: $_____**

☐ **PLEASE CHARGE TO MY CREDIT CARD.**

☐ Visa ☐ MasterCard ☐ AmEx ☐ Discover
☐ Diner's Club ☐ Eurocard ☐ JCB

Account # _____

Exp. Date_____

Signature_____

Prices in US dollars and subject to change without notice.

NAME_____

INSTITUTION_____

ADDRESS_____

CITY_____

STATE/ZIP_____

COUNTRY_____ COUNTY (NY residents only)_____

TEL_____ FAX_____

E-MAIL_____

May we use your e-mail address for confirmations and other types of information? ☐ Yes ☐ No
We appreciate receiving your e-mail address and fax number. Haworth would like to e-mail or fax special
discount offers to you, as a preferred customer. **We will never share, rent, or exchange your e-mail address
or fax number.** We regard such actions as an invasion of your privacy.

Order From Your Local Bookstore or Directly From
The Haworth Press, Inc.
10 Alice Street, Binghamton, New York 13904-1580 • USA
TELEPHONE: 1-800-HAWORTH (1-800-429-6784) / Outside US/Canada: (607) 722-5857
FAX: 1-800-895-0582 / Outside US/Canada: (607) 771-0012
E-mail to: orders@haworthpress.com

For orders outside US and Canada, you may wish to order through your local
sales representative, distributor, or bookseller.
For information, see http://haworthpress.com/distributors

(Discounts are available for individual orders in US and Canada only, not booksellers/distributors.)
PLEASE PHOTOCOPY THIS FORM FOR YOUR PERSONAL USE.
http://www.HaworthPress.com   BOF04